D0016642

Heart Disease

Heart Disease

Regis A. DeSilva

Biographies of Disease
Julie K. Silver, MD, Series Editor

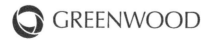

GREENWOOD

AN IMPRINT OF ABC-CLIO, LLC
Santa Barbara, California • Denver, Colorado • Oxford, England

Library of Congress Cataloging-in-Publication Data

DeSilva, Regis.
  Heart disease / Regis DeSilva.
    p. cm. — (Biographies of disease)
  Includes index.
    ISBN 978-0-313-37606-1 (hardback) — ISBN 978-0-313-37607-8 (ebook)
1. Heart—Diseases—Popular works. I. Title.

  RC672.D47   2013
  616.1'2—dc23   2012004998

ISBN: 978-0-313-37606-1
EISBN: 978-0-313-37607-8

17   16   15   14   13   1   2   3   4   5

This book is also available on the World Wide Web as an eBook.
Visit www.abc-clio.com for details.

Greenwood
An Imprint of ABC-CLIO, LLC

ABC-CLIO, LLC
130 Cremona Drive, P.O. Box 1911
Santa Barbara, California 93116–1911

This book is printed on acid-free paper (∞)

Manufactured in the United States of America

*This book is dedicated to my late parents
Mathew and Jessy DeSilva,
who made it all possible.*

Contents

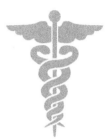

Series Foreword

Every disease has a story to tell: about how it started long ago and began to disable or even take the lives of its innocent victims, about the way it hurts us, and about how we are trying to stop it. In this Biographies of Disease series, the authors tell the stories of the diseases that we have come to know and dread.

The stories of these diseases have all of the components that make for great literature. There is incredible drama played out in real-life scenes from the past, present, and future. You'll read about how men and women of science stumbled trying to save the lives of those they aimed to protect. Turn the pages and you'll also learn about the amazing success of those who fought for health and won, often saving thousands of lives in the process.

If you don't want to be a health professional or research scientist now, when you finish this book you may think differently. The men and women in this book are heroes who often risked their own lives to save or improve ours. This is the biography of a disease, but it is also the story of real people who made incredible sacrifices to stop it in its tracks.

Julie K. Silver, MD
Assistant Professor, Harvard Medical School
Department of Physical Medicine and Rehabilitation

Acknowledgments

In writing this book, I owe a debt to several people. I wish to thank Professor Clifford Tabin, Chair of the Department of Genetics, Harvard Medical School; Dr. Deepak Srivastava, Wilma and Adeline Pirag Distinguished Professor of Pediatric and Developmental Cardiology and Director of the Gladstone Institute of Cardiovascular Disease, University of California, San Francisco; and Dr. James Lock, Alexander S. Nadas Professor of Pediatrics, Harvard Medical School and Cardiologist-in-Chief, Children's Hospital Medical Center, Boston. They were instrumental in providing useful information on specific aspects of new developments and treatments in cardiology.

Dr. Ernest Gervino, Associate Professor, Harvard Medical School and Director of the Exercise Stress Laboratory at Beth Israel Deaconess Medical Center, provided valuable input on exercise stress testing. Dr. Harvey Feigenbaum, Distinguished Professor, Indiana University School of Medicine, Indianapolis, provided me with information on the early history of echocardiography. Mr. Barouh V. Berkovits of Newton, Massachusetts, a senior engineer formerly at the American Optical Corporation and Medtronic Inc., and Igor F. Efimov, PhD, Lopata Distinguished Professor, Department of Biomedical Engineering, Washington University, St. Louis, Missouri alerted me to the early history of defibrillation in Russia.

Dr. Karim Benali of Abiomed, Inc. of Danvers, Massachusetts, provided information on artificial hearts and ventricular assist devices. I also owe a debt of gratitude to Professor Bernard Lown, my mentor who gave me a start at Harvard and influenced my own interest and research in ventricular fibrillation. Mr. John C. Bogle of Vanguard's Bogle Financial Markets Research Center, Malvern, Pennsylvania, very kindly shared his medical history and heart transplantation experience with me. Any errors in interpretation of information and reporting are mine alone.

I also wish to thank Brendan Ozawa-de Silva, D. Phil., of Emory University, Atlanta, Georgia, for reading parts of the manuscript for clarity and flow for a nonmedical reader. Ms. Marta Vilas Zarauza of Santiago de Compostela, Spain, was my Spanish-speaking reader who helped read the manuscript for understanding by someone whose native language is not English.

Finally, I want to thank Mr. Michael Nobel, my editor, who raised the manuscript to a higher level with his useful suggestions and editorial expertise to turn it into a better book.

Dr. Regis A. DeSilva
Physician, Cardiovascular Division
Beth Israel Deaconess Medical Center
Associate Professor of Medicine
Harvard Medical School
Boston, Massachusetts
USA

Introduction

The heart is a strange and mysterious organ that has mystical, romantic and magical associations. But the heart is also the cause of death for most people living in the West. And it is the only organ in the body capable of self-electrocution. This book tells the story of the heart, how it works and how it malfunctions. It also provides a narrative of how discoveries about the heart were made, how cures were found and a little about the people who made it possible.

Cardiology is the term used to describe the clinical specialty involving the study of the heart and great vessels and the medical conditions that affect them. The discipline of cardiology includes study of the normal physiological functioning of the heart and great vessels and the signs and symptoms of heart disease, diagnostic methods and tests used in heart disease and the treatment of such disorders. A *cardiologist* is a person who is a specialist in heart diseases and who diagnoses such diseases and treats them. A *cardiac surgeon* specializes in operating directly on the heart in an operating room.

The term *cardiovascular* system refers to the heart, great vessels, and the entire vascular system. The term is applied to describe someone as a *cardiovascular physician* (cardiologist) or as a *cardiovascular surgeon*. Typically, cardiologists and cardiac surgeons in the United States treat only the heart and blood vessels that are directly attached to the heart. Diseases of the *peripheral vascular system* (carotid arteries; aorta; and vessels in the abdomen, arms, and legs) are treated by *vascular surgeons*, who do not treat the heart. *Hypertension* (high blood pressure) is treated by either hypertension specialists or internists who are not necessarily cardiologists. In many countries there is a greater overlap between all these specialties, so this terminology may not apply in the same way as it does in the United States.

Cardiology and cardiac surgery have seen tremendous growth, especially in the past 50 years as new diagnostics and treatment have become available. These new discoveries and inventions have led to the prevention of fatal heart conditions, and there is clinical evidence that such treatments do indeed prolong life.

Cardiology is a very large area of research and clinical endeavor as it is the leading cause of death in the West. The field involves a wide range of specialists including epidemiologists, basic laboratory scientists, geneticists, clinical investigators, clinicians, nurses, and emergency medical technicians. It is fast becoming the most important disease in developing countries. This specialty also has the largest array of technological tools for diagnosis and treatment of any specialty in medicine. It often occupies the largest clinical footprint in any acute care hospital, and the cost of treatment imposes a high economic burden on society. However, since heart diseases often affect young and middle-aged people in their most productive years, early treatment may actually provide an economic benefit to a country.

I begin with an overview of the normal structure and function of the heart so that the reader's understanding is first grounded in basic anatomy and physiology. I have also provided a history of the evolution of thinking in cardiology over 2,000 years to show how discoveries were made, how new ideas have shaped progress, and how this made modern diagnostic methods and treatment possible. Next, the reader's attention is directed to the major diseases that affect the heart and great vessels, along with the signs and symptoms that occur when there is disordered function. Rather than describing the particular tests that are applied for each disease state, tests used to diagnose heart diseases are grouped together as a comprehensive review in one chapter. Because study of the heart is still an evolving science, the understanding of its disorders and the treatments applied are constantly changing. For this reason, I have taken the approach of not being prescriptive in writing this book. Rather, the book provides the essential information needed to make an informed decision that is suitable for a particular person in consultation with a specialist. Specific treatments for the conditions described must be discussed with one's own medical consultant in order to make an intelligent treatment choice.

In some chapters, I begin with a clinical narrative to illustrate some clinical concept or a technical point. These are actual patients I have treated in the past. However, details have been altered to preserve anonymity.

Risk factors for coronary artery disease are placed near the end of the book for two specific reasons. First, it is best to know the various afflictions of the heart before reading about risk factors for heart disease. Second, known risk factors generally refer only to coronary artery disease. Even then the known risk factors account only for about half of the prevalence of coronary artery disease. There are probably other undiscovered risk factors that we do not know about. I close with a futuristic look at what may come along in the diagnosis and treatment of heart disease. There is no way of predicting the future, just as no one could have predicted heart transplants or the discovery that some people are genetically programmed for some types of sudden death. At best this is just a guess of what may be in the future.

To make technical terms more understandable I have explained concepts in the text and have also provided a glossary of commonly used terms. The reader may find quite a bit of repetition of concepts already described in an earlier chapter. This was done to avoid losing the thread and having to go back to look up terms and concepts that were already referenced. I have also used abbreviations quite liberally, simply because they are commonly used in clinical medicine by doctors, nurses, and technicians, and one may as well get used to them.

This review cannot pretend to be comprehensive, but it should serve as scaffolding for further reading if it sparks your interest in cardiology. I have tried to describe the current state of the art and science rather than interpret research papers and scientific reports to avoid any personal bias I may have. Medical drug and device companies are mentioned without favor, and I have received no compensation from them. Sometimes, I have added cautionary notes when information is evolving or incomplete and, indeed, some information may have changed by the time the book goes to press. I have also tended to use the masculine pronoun for simplicity rather than to be exclusive. Similarly, I have used the term "doctor" in a generic sense when the person doing a test or rendering care may be a nurse or other caregiver, or one of the highly specialized technologists who are experts in their own right.

Some degree of simplification is inevitable in the interest of clarity when describing complex biological and technical systems or processes. A glossary of useful technical terms is provided to aid readers in the accepted definition of commonly used terms in cardiology. At the end of some of the chapters, a number of useful references and websites are provided for the reader interested in original source material. Many of the websites contain current recommendations for major cardiovascular conditions from the National Heart, Lung and Blood Institute; the American Heart Association; the American College of Cardiology; the Centers for Disease Control; and other sources. These sources can answer questions that may arise relating to specific recommendations for various diseases that are described in this book.

The information in the book and the original sources provided are rendered as objectively as possible. My hope is that this information will help people with heart disease to make informed decisions about their health.

Dr. Regis A. DeSilva
Associate Professor of Medicine
Harvard Medical School
Physician, Cardiovascular Division
Beth Israel Deaconess Medical Center
Boston, Massachusetts

1

History of Cardiology

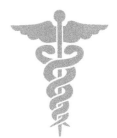

> The poets did well to conjoin music and medicine in Apollo: because
> the office of medicine is but to tune this curious harp of man's body
> and to reduce it to harmony.
>
> —*Francis Bacon (1561–1626)*

In nearly all cultures, religion, magic, and healing have been inextricably intertwined. Healers were often seen as high priests or magicians, or a combination of both, privy to esoteric knowledge that they guarded jealously. Practitioners of the healing arts were not timid about invoking a higher authority to effect cures and to enhance their own power. They claimed to have special knowledge, and most of it was kept secret, though much knowledge about health and disease was largely erroneous. Such secrecy enhanced the power of the healer over the afflicted person, though it is likely that this power had the healing effect of a powerful placebo. Early medical practice was thus often clouded by a combination of various belief systems, religion, magical rituals, and even touches of Satanism.

In only a minority of cases did practitioners actually dissect bodies to examine diseased structures, or prepare themselves for their craft by studying human anatomy. In even fewer cases was there the study of physiology to understand the inner workings of the organs of the body. Many of the treatments prescribed were, therefore, unfounded on scientific logic.

Of all the internal organs, the mysteriously beating human heart has had the greatest emotional and mystical significance. In ancient times, the heart was believed to have spiritual and even divine attributes. Both the Old Testament (the Jewish Bible) and the Talmud make reference to the heart, which is referred to as *lev* or *levav*. There are anatomical descriptions of the heart in these texts that probably date from the fifth to the second centuries BCE. In the Upanishads, the Hindu texts that date back to about 300 BCE, the description of the heart includes its covering (the pericardium), proving recognition of its anatomical structure.

The persistence of esoteric knowledge related to bodily function and health is also seen in alchemy, astrology, anthroposophy, Christian Science, Theosophy, and Rosicrucianism. Even in more modern times, there are strong connections between religious beliefs and the heart. One such example is the cult of the Sacred Heart in French Catholic devotional life. Systematic studies of the heart and its physiological functions had to await the passage of several more centuries. The Renaissance, spanning from the 14th to the 17th centuries, began in Italy and spread to the rest of Europe. This movement saw a resurgence of artistic creativity and scientific investigation that opened the way for a systematic study of the heart and circulation.

EARLY CONCEPTS OF THE CIRCULATION

The ancient Egyptians did the first human anatomical examinations because anatomical dissection was essential to the practice of embalming the dead. In the third century BCE, Alexandria was the seat of Egyptian and Hellenistic culture, patronized by the pharaoh Ptolemy I Soter (367–283 BCE). The establishment of a medical school in Alexandria further promoted the study of anatomy. However, despite the ancient Egyptians' apparently advanced medical and surgical knowledge, the role of the heart in the circulation of blood was not well understood at the time.

The discoveries of what are now known as the Edwin Smith Papyrus and the Ebers Papyrus were essential to our understanding of how the Egyptians studied anatomy and prescribed medical treatments. The Smith Papyrus, acquired by Edwin Smith in Thebes in 1862, is dated from around 3000–1600 BCE, or at least 1,200 years before Hippocrates. Some authorities believe it to be derived from the work of Imhotep, the first known physician. The Smith Papyrus deals largely with anatomy and surgical trauma but also correlates the pumping action of the heart with the pulse. This document describes the heart as being the center of a system from which all blood vessels radiate to the rest of the body.

The Ebers Papyrus, produced about 1550 BCE, or roughly 1,500 years after the Smith Papyrus, was acquired also in Thebes by the German Egyptologist Georg Ebers in 1872. The Ebers Papyrus is one of the most important early documents in medicine, and contains "A Treatise on the Heart." This work also places the heart as the center of circulation and noted that it was attached to all major organs by blood vessels. The heart was therefore considered to be the center of the blood supply as it provided blood to the rest of the body. The circulatory system was also thought to carry other fluids such as urine, tears, and semen to the heart from other organs.

The ancient Egyptians' views were mirrored by the ancient Greeks, as articulated by Aristotle who lived from 384 BCE to 322 BCE. Both Aristotle and Hippocrates (c. 460–370 BCE) considered the heart as the source of innate heat, which was a view that persisted for almost two thousand years. The Egyptians believed that the heart, rather than the brain, was the source of human wisdom, emotions, and memory, and the seat of the soul and personality. It was through the heart that God spoke, giving the ancient Egyptians knowledge of God and God's will. For this reason, it was considered the most important of the body's organs.

Galen of Pergamon (c. 130–200 CE), the great Greek physician, disagreed with the prevailing view. He dissected a variety of animals and practiced very daring surgery on the brain, the eye, and the heart. He viewed the brain as the seat of reason, the heart as the seat of emotion, and the liver the seat of passion. Furthermore, Galen believed there were two kinds of blood: *nutritive* blood made by the liver and *vital* blood made by the heart and pumped through arteries. The heart was a source of heat and the blood cooled as it circulated. He assumed that blood traversed the ventricular septum, from one side of the heart to the other, through tiny pores. The lungs, with the movement of air through them, had a fanning and cooling function on the heart.

Galen's views were widely taught well into the 15th and 16th centuries. Despite Galenic misconceptions and frequent references to the Almighty, some progress was made by anatomists of the era. Leonardo da Vinci (1452–1519) made detailed and accurate dissections of the heart that unfortunately were never published. Anatomists and scholars, such as Berengario (1460–1630), described the various chambers of the heart. Other noted scholars, namely Vesalius (1513–1564), Servetus (1511–1553), and Cesalpino (1524–1603), further advanced understanding of the anatomy of the heart. Servetus, a Spaniard, was the first European to describe the circulation of blood through the lungs.

Ibn al-Nafis (1213–1288), an Arab physician, was actually the first person to describe the pulmonary circulation before Servetus. He was also the first to challenge the long-held view of the Galen school that blood could pass through the cardiac septum via microscopic pores. Al-Nafis believed that blood that reached the heart passed through the lungs, so that there must be small communications between the pulmonary artery and the pulmonary vein. This important deduction preceded the discovery of pulmonary capillaries, which connect arteries to veins, by Marcello Malpighi (1628–1694) 400 years later.

These contradictory and confusing discoveries laid the shaky foundations for the work of William Harvey, on whom it fell to clarify how the heart and circulation really worked.

DISCOVERY OF THE CIRCULATION

The circulation of blood was a mystery that took over 2,000 years of scientific thinking to unravel. This long process may have been due to the curiously mystical nature of the heart, even within scientific circles. A sacred and somewhat godly view of the heart, as I have described, impeded scientific examination of how it actually functioned as a mechanical pump.

In the early 17th century, both René Descartes (1596–1650) and William Harvey (1578–1657) studied the heart and came to very different conclusions. They were aware by this time that the brain was the seat of neurological activity, and understood that the heart was responsible for the circulation of blood. Descartes's view was that the heart was a furnace-like organ heating blood that rose to the brain, where it cooled, and then descended to the right atrium of the heart to be recycled. This schema obviated the need for blood to cross over from the right side of the heart to the left side, via pores, since no such pores could be found.

It was William Harvey who, in 1628 in his book *Exercitatio Anatomica de Motu Cordis et Sanguinis in Animalibus* ("An Anatomical Exercise on the Motion of the Heart and Blood in Living Beings"), captured the essential mechanical workings of the heart. He experimented on birds, reptiles, and small mammals, making meticulous measurements on how blood left the heart and how, after traveling around the body, returned to it again. Harvey was a punctilious man and he showed the heart and circulation were made up of two interlocking systems: the *systemic circulation* and the *pulmonary circulation*.

Harvey explained how blood was pumped out of the left side of the heart and into the arterial system to nourish the rest of the body. This part of the circulation is called the *systemic circulation*. After delivering oxygen to the body, venous blood returns to the right side of the heart, where it is pumped this time to the lungs. Blood is oxygenated in the lungs and is then returned to the left side of the heart to be pumped out, yet again, to the rest of the body. This circuit is referred to as the *pulmonary circulation*. He laid down the principles for the fundamental physiology of the heart by making volumetric measurements today known as *stroke volume* and *cardiac output*. Descartes, Jean Riolan, Ole Worm, Marin Mersenne, and a motley collection of other part-time scientists scoffed at this idea, though they had absolutely no scientific evidence to refute Harvey's exposition.

Harvey was ridiculed and thoroughly derided at the time, but his theory was later confirmed and has held true to this day. More importantly, it opened a new era of scientific thinking grounded on observation and experimentation.

The ancient Greeks, the Egyptians, and the Europeans, who revived Neoplatonism during the Renaissance, often invoked idiosyncratic explanations for natural phenomena by references to the Divine or the will of anthropomorphic gods. Harvey took a *rationalistic* approach that is reminiscent of Thales, the pre-Socratic philosopher who rejected divine or supernatural explanations. Rationalism appeals to reason as the source of knowledge or for the justification of a particular position. Harvey therefore occupies the important space between pre-modern and modern scientific thinking in physiology and medicine. This is why Harvey, after Charles Darwin, is the second most cited scientist in the biological sciences.

DEVELOPMENT OF QUANTITATIVE METHODS IN CARDIOLOGY

As noted above, Harvey laid the foundations for quantitative thinking in medical physiology. His work allowed the emergence of a scientific approach, not only in cardiology, but in biological physiology. His work was groundbreaking as it was key to the development of a new approach to biological explanations. He did this by formulating a hypothesis, careful experimentation, and repeated measurements for verification, rather than by merely postulating theories that were unproven. Harvey's approach was truly innovative, and it firmly established the scientific method in the biological sciences for future research.

The next major step in cardiac physiology came in the person of another Englishman, Reverend Stephen Hales (1677–1761). In the expansive manner of scientists of the day, Hales was a Doctor of Divinity, a noted botanist, and a keen, energetic student of physiology. In his parsonage stable in 1727, Hales measured blood pressure directly by inserting a glass tube into the carotid artery in the neck of a white mare while it was forcibly held down. The glass tube was 12 feet, 9 inches (3.9 meters) long, and the horse's blood rose within it to a height of 9 feet,

6 inches (2.9 meters). Hales began his blood pressure measurement experiments around 1706 and reported his findings in a book called *Haemastaticks* in 1733.

A more practical, safer, and less gruesome noninvasive method for measuring blood pressure in humans was devised by the French doctor and physiologist Étienne-Jules Marey (1830–1904) in 1857. Marey, incidentally, also devised high-speed cinematography for scientific studies that later led to the making of movies for entertainment by the Lumière Brothers in the 1890s. In the 1950s, cinematography would be applied to filming the heart using X-rays during cardiac catheterization.

Marey devised a wrist sphygmograph that was later improved upon by Robert Ellis Dudgeon (1820–1904) in England in 1881, with a device known as a kymograph. The pulse at the wrist caused a metal strip to move a stylus, transmitting a record of the pulse onto smoked paper affixed to a rotating drum. The kymograph traces a wave-like line, which represents a record of blood pressure and pulse over time. In 1881, Siegfried von Basch (1837–1905), a professor in experimental pathology at the University of Vienna, developed a similar instrument. It was the sphygmomanometer, a portable noninvasive instrument for measuring blood pressure.

The Italian internist and pediatrician Scipione Riva-Rocci (1863–1937) invented a sphygmomanometer to measure blood pressure in 1896 using an inkwell, some copper piping, a bicycle tube, and a vertical glass column containing mercury. An inflatable arm cuff was used to compress the brachial artery in the arm so that blood pressure could be measured at the elbow. The mercury manometer was used in the United States until 2000, but it has since largely been replaced by aneroid and digital blood pressure devices, though it is still used widely elsewhere in the world.

Since blood pressure has a wave-like pulsating form, it has two descriptive values: *systolic blood pressure* and *diastolic blood pressure*. The systolic pressure is the higher number (e.g., 120 millimeters of mercury); and the lower number is the diastolic pressure (e.g., 70 millimeters of mercury), denoting the lower limit of blood pressure. Normal blood pressure is not a fixed number but fluctuates between the systolic and the diastolic pressures. Blood pressure is therefore described, using the numbers from the example cited above, as being 120/70 millimeters of mercury (or mmHg).

It was not possible to measure the lower number accurately using an external noninvasive method until 1921, when a Russian physician in St. Petersburg, Nikolai Korotkoff (1874–1920), succeeded in doing so. He essentially devised the method still used today by inflating an arm cuff with air to compress the brachial artery in the arm. Listening to the artery at the elbow just below the cuff with a stethoscope, Korotkoff heard various types of sounds caused by the pulsating flow of blood on gradually releasing cuff pressure by deflating it by releasing a valve. The sounds are now eponymously called *Korotkoff sounds*. These sounds provide accurate estimates of both systolic and diastolic blood pressure that are useful for clinical measurement.

THE CARDIAC EXAMINATION AND INVENTION OF THE STETHOSCOPE

Palpation of the pulse and the heartbeat has been done for over 3,000 years. Chinese medical practitioners thought the pulse to be very important in diagnosing various medical conditions. Other than taking the pulse, and looking at, smelling, and tasting the urine, many physicians in Europe, until the 19th century, did little else. So-called Piss Prophets would claim that every disease could be diagnosed and treated by a thorough examination of the urine, even without seeing the patient! Those who bothered to examine patients would perform only the most cursory of physical examinations using methods of direct observation and palpation with their hands. The heart was sometimes examined by direct auscultation, where doctors listened to the heart with their ears applied to the chest, often protected by a silk handkerchief carried for that purpose. It is not clear what exactly they were listening to, or what the sounds meant to them, since they had only a vague idea what information such an examination might reveal.

Diseases of the heart can impact many organs, and clues may be hidden in distant parts of the body, such as the limbs, the skin, and the eyes. To make an accurate cardiac diagnosis, a complete examination is necessary not only of the heart but also of the lungs, other internal organs, and indeed the whole body. Detailed clinical examination of the heart and lungs was made possible by the invention of the stethoscope by René-Théophile-Hyacinthe Laënnec (1781–1826) in 1818 in Paris. He was consulted on a rather corpulent young female patient and found auscultation embarrassing and almost impossible due to her ample breasts.

While working at the Hôpital Necker, Laënnec had seen some young children playing near the Louvre, listening to the ends of long pieces of timber that transmitted the sounds of pin scratches while listening through a hollow stick. The next day, he rolled up a quire of paper, tied it with string, and listened to his patient's chest with it. To his surprise he heard the heart sounds more distinctly and more loudly than by direct auscultation.

In his woodworking shop he milled a 25 centimeter by 2.5 centimeter hollow wooden cylinder that he used to listen to the chest sounds of his patients. He later modified this cylinder to have detachable parts to be carried easily. Laënnec called his instrument the *stethoscope*. As it was used to auscultate the heart using only one ear, it was called a *monaural* ("one ear") stethoscope.

He described and named the various lung sounds and heart sounds he heard in different disease conditions. Physicians still use the same descriptive terms today (e.g., *râles, rhonchi*) for various sounds heard through the stethoscope in conditions such as in congestive heart failure or pneumonia. Laënnec presented his findings to the Académie de Médecine in Paris in 1818, and the following year, he published his book *De l'Auscultation Médiate* ("On Mediate Auscultation"). Initially, as with many new innovations in medicine, neither his new instrument nor his book were received with favor.

Progressive improvements by other inventors have produced the *binaural* ("two ear") stethoscope with two earpieces that we use today. The stethoscope is not only indispensible in modern medical practice, but it has also famously become the hallmark of a physician. With its use, a skilled and artful physician can often make a surprisingly accurate diagnosis of many heart conditions. Such conditions may range from valve abnormalities and congenital heart disease to congestive heart failure.

The medical history and the physical examination together form the basis for the practice of medicine. Since heart diseases may have effects on other organs and may even affect the skin, eyes, and limbs, a full physical examination is necessary. Both the history and physical examination are indispensible to establish an initial diagnosis before specialized tests can be done in order to make a final diagnosis. As modern tests and treatments are often extremely expensive, it is essential to make a well-honed provisional diagnosis before embarking on an appropriate series of initial diagnostic tests.

RESEARCH IN CARDIAC PHYSIOLOGY

Diseases of the heart were known to cause early death, and often very rapidly. However, not much was known about how death actually occurred in heart disease. Anatomical study alone of the body and its organs is not sufficient to treat diseases. Often such detailed examinations were possible only after death, until the advent of new diagnostic methods in the 20th century. A physician needs to know how the body actually works; and when something goes wrong, how to correct it. The study of the normal workings of the body is called *physiology*. The study of diseases of various organs is called *pathology*. When organs malfunction as a result of disease, this altered state of function is called *pathophysiology*.

Investigations into the physiology of the heart and its mechanical function saw a golden age in the 19th century, led by two giants of cardiac research: Michael

Foster (1836–1907), in England, and Carl Ludwig (1816–1895), in Germany. Through the doors of their two laboratories passed a number of famous physiologists who researched the heart, brain, kidneys, and nervous system.

One of the great mysteries of the heart at that time was how it was capable of rhythmic action, and how it could continue beating even when taken out of the chest. This discovery had already been made by the great Galen of Pergamon several centuries earlier. The idea of the heart as an electromechanically coupled organ began to emerge as a result of research in the 19th century. A rough analogy would be an internal combustion engine that needs an electrical system to make it fire and function mechanically. Research done in the laboratories of both Foster and Ludwig established that though the heart and the brain were closely linked, the heart could also beat independently of the nervous system. Scientists at both laboratories also worked on the electrical system of the heart. They showed that this internal wiring, called the *conduction system of the heart,* is the component that keeps the organ beating rhythmically.

One of the amazing discoveries made in Ludwig's laboratory in 1850 was that there was a chaotic rhythm called *ventricular fibrillation* that could kill an animal. This rhythm could be induced by an electrical current and caused death by electrocution within a few minutes. At the time, this arrhythmia was largely a laboratory curiosity, but it led to a new and exciting area of research.

In 1889, John MacWilliam (1857–1937), a Scottish physician and physiologist, after experimenting on animals, deduced accurately that ventricular fibrillation was the rhythm primarily responsible for the sudden collapse and death in humans. He based this theory on the newly emerging field of evolutionary biology. Charles Darwin had published his book *On the Origin of Species* in 1859, and the introduction of the concept of evolution spurred a new direction of thinking in science. MacWilliam saw a phylogenetic similarity between the electrical behavior of hearts progressing from fish to frog to man. He logically extended his experiments on ventricular fibrillation in lower animals to humans, surmising that this arrhythmia was the cause of *sudden death.* MacWilliam's theory was proved to be correct in the latter half of the 20th century. Doctors discovered in the 1960s that sudden death was, indeed, often due to ventricular fibrillation. This was supported by the examination of electrocardiograms taken from people who had collapsed from cardiac arrest.

The electrocardiogram had actually not yet been invented when Ludwig and MacWilliam performed their animal experiments. Ludwig used a kymograph, a mechanical instrument of his own invention, to track the functions of the heart. As described earlier, the kymograph had a rotating drum with smoked paper on its surface. A movable stylus attached by a piece of string to the beating heart traced a pattern on the paper as the heart underwent changes in rate and rhythm in response to various stimuli. Paul Cranefield, a Rockefeller University electrophysiologist, later compared the invention of this instrument to that of the telescope in astronomy, as it opened vast new vistas for the quantitative exploration of the heartbeat.

Using the kymograph in 1913, George Ralph Mines (1886–1914) discovered one of the keystone concepts in cardiac electrophysiology called the *vulnerable period*. During a very brief period in the cardiac cycle, an external stimulus such as an electrical pulse or a physical blow to the heart (e.g., a baseball hitting the chest wall) can trigger ventricular fibrillation and cause sudden death. The discovery that ventricular fibrillation caused sudden death led to a search for a way to stop ventricular fibrillation once it has begun. The story of how people could actually be resuscitated from almost certain death using electrical defibrillation is described in later chapters.

DEVELOPMENT OF ELECTROPHYSIOLOGY

Early Experimental Work

William Gilbert (1544–1603), physician to Queen Elizabeth I in England, studied magnetism and the properties of static electricity produced by rubbing amber. He coined the word *electricity* from the Latin word *electricus*, meaning "like amber." Amber is called *elektron* in Greek, from which the word *electron* is derived. Gilbert published his magnum opus in 1600, and in his classic book *De Magnete*, he concluded that the earth was a giant magnet. This explained why the magnetic lodestone compass always pointed North and South. He also thought electricity and magnetism were somehow related to one another.

In the late 1700s and early 1800s, many experimenters like Benjamin Franklin in the United States, Hans Christian Oersted in Denmark, André-Marie Ampère in France, Georg Ohm in Germany, and Michael Faraday in England were experimenting with the physics of electricity. They collectively created some of the terminology and measurement units (the *oersted*, the *ampere* and the *ohm*) we use in electricity today.

Bioelectricity has been known since the time of the Egyptians in 2750 BCE. It was recognized later by the ancient Greeks, who rediscovered the electrogenic properties of electric eels, catfish, and torpedo rays. These fish have electric organs that are, basically, thousands of stacked electrical cells that can charge and store electricity like a battery. The stored electricity can be discharged at will to stun or kill prey, or when the fish is threatened. Such fish can generate 1 ampere and 500 volts in the case of eels, and 30 amperes and up to 200 volts in rays. These levels of electricity are enough to kill an adult human.

Electrophysiology is the study of electrical activity occurring in living tissue. Like many biological experiments, electrical studies in animals started with frogs and toads, as they are plentiful and easily captured. The Italian physician Luigi Galvani (1737–1798), from Bologna, accidentally discovered that static electricity generated by the instruments he was working with caused a dead frog's leg to twitch. Galvani called this kind of animation *animal electricity* in 1791.

His Italian contemporary Alessandro Volta (1745–1827) named this effect *galvanism*. Even today, we speak of people being *galvanized* when they become energized into action. Basically, Galvani "energized" his dead frog's leg because his instruments, made up of two different kinds of metal, produced a charge that translated into an electrical current. This observation became the basis for an electric cell made of two metals such as copper (*positive pole*) and zinc (*negative pole*) that generate an electric current. Volta—for whom the term *volt* is named—stacked piles of such cells into what we now call a *battery*. Negatively charged electrons flow from the negative to the positive pole, so that the directional flow of current is from the positive to the negative pole.

Galvani's work influenced Carol Mateucci (1811–1868), professor of physics in Pisa, who studied bioelectric phenomena in frogs. He in turn influenced Emil du Bois-Reymond (1818–1896), the French-German physician and today considered the father of electrophysiology. His studies on the biology of electrical phenomena in nerve cells led to the discovery the *action potential*, a basic concept in bioelectricity.

Invention of the Electrocardiogram

Bioelectric phenomena in living cells, where living cells generate *electrical potentials*, are similar to the way electrical batteries work. A bioelectric current is caused by a flow of ions (i.e., electrically charged atoms or molecules) across a permeable cell membrane. One side is negatively charged and the other positively charged, and the ions involved, also known as electrolytes, are typically sodium, potassium, and calcium. Cell membrane activity pumps the ions across the membrane, so that a charge of around 50 millivolts is maintained in the resting state. Either spontaneously or whenever stimulated, cells can depolarize, and the rapid flow of ions across the cell membrane creates what is known as an *action potential*. Many cardiac cells are capable of spontaneously discharging electrical impulses to create rhythmic action and contraction of the heart.

The studies by the Englishmen Alan Hodgkin (1914–1998) and Andrew Huxley (1917–2012) on the giant squid axon led to a detailed understanding of how nerve cells function to generate electrical activity. They were awarded the Nobel Prize in Physiology or Medicine along with the Australian John Eccles (1903–1997) in 1963 for their seminal studies on the action potential. Their studies shed light on how the heart functioned as an electrical organ at a cellular level.

One of the problems faced by early experimenters was that such electrical activity is invisible and no devices existed until the 19th century for the documentation of electrical events. The generation of electricity by animals and the action of electricity on living creatures could only be studied by the effects they produced. The clinical question was: how do we measure the electrical activity of the intact heart in a living human being?

Before the invention of the electrocardiogram (EKG), the heartbeat could only be studied by its mechanical movement as it contracted and relaxed using a kymograph, as described earlier. While the electric motor invented by Michael Faraday (1791–1867) produced large currents that could be easily measured, the heart muscle and nerve cells produced barely perceptible currents that required very sensitive instruments.

The EKG was first recorded by Étienne-Jules Marey in Paris in 1876 using a mercury capillary electrometer. The electrometer was invented by fellow Frenchman, Gabriel Lippman, in 1872. A column of mercury in the glass capillary moved up and down when it detected a tiny flow of electrical current passing through it. By using this device in London in 1887, Augustus Waller (1856–1922) recorded the electrical activity of the human heart indirectly with electrodes attached to the surface of the body. This discovery led to the ultimate invention of the EKG about 20 years later.

The EKG was developed into a practical clinical diagnostic tool by the Dutch physician and experimental physiologist Willem Einthoven (1860–1927). He invented a string galvanometer attached to a mirror that deflected upon detecting a current. This instrument, named for Galvani, can measure the extremely small currents generated by the heart. The movements of the mirror were amplified by projecting a light beam falling on it across a darkened room. He photographed the movements using a moving sheet of photographic film that, when developed, showed an EKG tracing.

Einthoven positioned electrical leads on three of the limbs of the body (right and left arms and right leg), along with one ground lead on the left leg. (An electrical lead is an insulated wire with electrodes at the end of it.) The lines connecting the three limb leads form the "Einthoven triangle," made up of Lead I (right arm to left arm), Lead II (right arm to left leg), and Lead III (left arm to left leg). These standard leads are still used today to record the EKG. Subsequently, three augmented limb leads (aVR, aVL, and aVF) were added by Emanuel Goldberger in 1942, and six additional chest leads (V1 through V6) were added in 1944 to the system by Frank N. Wilson. The modern EKG system used today therefore has a total of 12 leads. By looking at the heart from 12 different positions, it is possible to create a sort of electrical map of the heart. Einthoven also gave the names P, Q, R, S, and T to the waves of the EKG, following the Descartes convention for naming points on mathematical diagrams. The events related to the electrical waves of the EKG and how they represent activity of the heart are discussed in detail in chapter 8.

The EKG tracing today is recorded on graph paper marked with a grid that shows time in milliseconds on the X-axis and voltage in millivolts on the Y-axis. These measurements allow interpretation of events in two dimensions: the strength of the electrical impulse in millivolts and the time an impulse takes to travel through the heart. These measurements help in making clinical diagnoses. Einthoven won the Nobel Prize in Medicine or Physiology in 1924 for producing a clinically useful EKG device and for his early work on electrocardiography.

Clinical Applications of the EKG

In the 1960s and 1970s, EKGs taken during prehospital resuscitation proved that sudden death in heart disease was most often due to ventricular fibrillation, as predicted previously by John MacWilliam in 1889. The EKG is now used to diagnose various other rhythm disturbances and to help diagnose myocardial infarction. When diagnosed at an early stage, this helps salvage the heart from further damage during a heart attack.

In the 1960s, in the United States, Europe, and Australia, patients with myocardial infarction and unstable angina were clustered together in a specialized area in the hospital called *coronary care units* (CCU). The CCU allowed continuous monitoring of the heart rhythm, regular observations of blood pressure, and rapid response to emergencies such as cardiac arrest or an acute loss of blood pressure. The staff was specially trained in cardiac resuscitation and defibrillation and in the use of specialized drugs and instruments such as balloon pumps. This rapid response team allowed for early interventions to be performed rapidly during cardiac emergencies.

The EKG could also be monitored continuously in the free-living person with a compact recorder attached by electrical leads to the chest. This device was originally a cassette tape recorder, but today a digital recorder is used. Such a device allowed doctors to analyze the EKG made over a long period of time and make a diagnosis if a rhythm disturbance was suspected.

Exercise stress testing with continuous EKG monitoring was developed in the 1950s and 1960s. These tests done on a stationary bicycle or a treadmill became the standard method to make a diagnosis of coronary heart disease. Continuous EKG monitoring is invaluable in diagnosis and treatment under a variety of circumstances where the heart is judged to be at risk. For example, EKG monitoring is used routinely during surgery in the operating room, regardless of the type of surgery being done.

The Artificial Pacemaker

After the invention of the EKG, it was apparent that following heart attacks and during cardiac surgery, the heart could become abnormally slow and even stop. Efforts were made to study if electrical stimulation could be applied to keep it beating. John MacWilliam had already noted in 1899 that external electrical stimuli delivered about 70 times a minute could keep the heart beating effectively after it had stopped.

Several early investigators invented devices to keep the heart beating. Though it is difficult to imagine it today, they declined to publicize their attempts to revive stopped hearts due to negative publicity and fears about interfering with nature, and indeed, even with life itself. For example, the early efforts by Mark Lidwell and Edgar Booth in Sydney, Australia (1926), and Albert and Charles Hyman in New York (1932), were abandoned due to fears of public disapprobation. In both instances, electrical pacemakers were successfully constructed and deployed, but experimentation was halted. With the Sydney experimenters, a stillborn infant was successfully revived in 1928 at the Royal Alfred Hospital, and the child survived long term. Albert Hyman coined the term "artificial pacemaker," which is a term we still use today.

In the 1950s, John Hopps and W. G. Bigelow in Toronto designed an external pacemaker using vacuum tube circuits. Paul Zoll (1911–1999) in Boston also designed a pacemaker, but it was still very large by today's standards. The Canadians used alternating current (AC) power and Zoll used a large rechargeable battery. These devices were bulky and not very practical as they were often powered from AC sockets. Besides, they could cause painful shocks and ran the risk of causing ventricular fibrillation. If the patient's heart recovered spontaneously, the pacemaker could be disconnected and the patient discharged from hospital.

The invention of the transistor dramatically changed the field of electronics. J. L. Lillenfeld (1882–1963) patented a transistor in 1930 in the United States, but it did not immediately see application in medical instrumentation. John Bardeen, Walter Brattain, and William Shockley patented the modern transistor in 1947, for which they received the Nobel Prize in Physics for their work in 1956. This invention allowed the miniaturization of electrical devices to a remarkable degree, so that these devices can now be implanted into the body.

C. Walton Lillehei (1918–1999) was responsible for bringing the issue to the forefront. As a pioneering cardiac surgeon in Minnesota, he performed many innovative operations on adults with congenital heart disease. A result of surgical trauma was a condition called *heart block,* which caused slowing or stoppage of the heart and could occur during or after surgery. In 1957, ominously on Halloween, one of Lillehei's pediatric patients with a pacemaker died as a result of a massive power blackout in Minnesota and Wisconsin. Lillehei needed a battery-powered pacemaker to keep the heart beating, and he recruited the talents of Earl Bakken (b. 1924), an electronic engineer. Bakken invented a compact external transistorized pacemaker based on the circuitry of a metronome he saw in *Popular Mechanics*. Within a few weeks, he delivered to Lillehei a book-sized, yet operational, battery-powered pacemaker.

The first pacemaker implantation was done on Arne Larsson at the Karolinska Institute in Sweden in 1958. It failed after a few hours and the second pacemaker failed after two days. The patient, who underwent repeated pacemaker implants, went on to live to be 86, dying in 2001.

Subsequently, Wilson Greatbach (1919–2011) invented a mercury battery-powered, implantable pacemaker that was inserted into a patient by William Chardack in Buffalo in 1960. Greatbach later invented a lithium iodide battery that has since become standard as it can last as long as 14 years. The Chardack-Greatbach pacemaker, as it was known, was licensed to Medtronic Inc., in 1961. Today, 3 million people live with implanted pacemakers, and 600,000 pacemakers are implanted every year. Bakken and his brother-in-law, Palmer Hermundslie, founded Medtronic in his garage in 1949. Today, it is the leading medical device company in the world with a market capitalization of $43 billion.

MYOCARDIAL INFARCTION AND SUDDEN CARDIAC DEATH

It was in 1912 that James Herrick (1861–1954), a Chicago physician, proposed that a heart attack (*myocardial infarction*) was due to coronary thrombosis.

He suggested that the coronary arteries feeding the heart with blood and oxygen could become clogged with clots, thus causing a heart attack. His hypothesis has been found to be largely true as fresh clots, often on a ruptured cholesterol plaque, are responsible for a myocardial infarction.

Ventricular fibrillation (VF) occurs suddenly and is impossible to predict from the resting EKG. In fact, it is extremely difficult to predict it all. In the 1940s, the Consolidated Edison Company, which supplied electricity to New York, became concerned because its linemen were getting accidentally electrocuted. The cause of death was ventricular fibrillation. The company contacted William Bennett Kouwenhoven (1886–1975), an engineer at the Physics Laboratory at Johns Hopkins University in Baltimore, to come up with a solution. Kouwenhoven and his colleagues rediscovered the fact that electrical currents, while causing VF, could also be used to reverse it as well.

While experimenting with animals, they also laid down the basis for cardiopulmonary resuscitation. In 1960, they found that external chest compressions could cause blood pressure to increase by pumping blood out of the heart into the circulation. However, these findings were in fact rediscoveries, as in the late 1800s, John MacWilliam had already discovered the basis for cardiopulmonary resuscitation. MacWilliam had even found that he could pace the heart with electrical stimulation. The Swiss scientists Jean-Louis Prévost and Frederic Battelli had also already discovered around 1899 that small currents caused VF and larger currents terminated it.

Claude Beck, a surgeon, used an AC defibrillator in 1947 in a human for the first time to terminate VF. He operated on a 14-year-old boy with congenital heart disease, and while closing the chest, the patient developed ventricular fibrillation. He re-opened the chest and successfully applied current directly to the heart with a defibrillator he designed. The boy was revived and made a full recovery.

Early defibrillators in the United States used AC, but soon proved to be unreliable. These devices could actually provoke ventricular fibrillation again after first terminating it, due to the effects of a long duration pulse of AC on the heart. In the mid-1930s, Naum L. Gurvich, in Moscow, invented the basic circuitry used today in the electrical defibrillator. Gurvich had designed a defibrillator that delivered a single direct current (DC) capacitor discharge. He later added an inductance coil to dampen the electrical pulse. This addition to the circuit prolongs the pulse duration to five milliseconds and reduces damage to the heart caused by a large electrical discharge. These DC defibrillators were in use in Soviet Union hospitals in the early 1950s, well before they were used in the West.

Electricity could be used to terminate other arrhythmias, such as atrial fibrillation and ventricular tachycardia. However, discharges delivered randomly in the cardiac cycle could accidentally lead to ventricular fibrillation. The discovery of vulnerable period by George Ralph Mines in 1913 led to a modification of the defibrillator for terminating cardiac arrhythmias other than ventricular fibrillation.

The addition of a timing device to the electrical circuitry of a DC defibrillator by Bernard Lown and Barouh Berkovits around 1960 allowed the delivery of a current during a safe period during the cardiac cycle on the EKG. Troublesome arrhythmias could be terminated using electric current timed in such a way as to avoid triggering of fibrillation by a pulse falling on the T-wave of the EKG. This modification of the defibrillator was called the *cardioverter* and the method itself was named *cardioversion* by Lown. Cardioversion allowed the rapid treatment of ventricular tachycardia and atrial arrhythmias for which there was no other effective treatment at that time.

Today, defibrillators are routinely used in advanced life support (ALS) in hospitals and in ambulances. Automatic external defibrillators (AED) are now available in public places such as shopping malls, stadiums, airports, and airplanes. An implantable defibrillator was devised by Morton Mower and Michel Mirowski (1924–1990). The first implantation took place in 1980 at Johns Hopkins Hospital in Baltimore, Maryland. Today, automatic implantable cardioverter-defibrillators (AICD) are also capable of functioning as pacemakers. Defibrillators are commonly implanted to prevent sudden death after cardiac arrest or in patients at high risk for this condition.

MODERN CARDIAC DIAGNOSTIC METHODS

Practical approaches for the treatment of both myocardial infarction and rhythm disturbances had to await the development of other diagnostic methods. In 1929, the German physician Werner Forssmann (1904–1979), after anesthetizing his own arm, passed a urinary catheter into his own heart via a vein. When a nurse objected to this dangerous experiment, he tied her to an operating table and proceeded nonetheless. He then walked down a flight of stairs to the radiology department and took an X-ray of his heart that showed the tip of the catheter was located in the right atrium. He was sacked from his job and had to continue his work as a urologist rather than in cardiology. However, in 1956, he was awarded the Nobel Prize in Physiology or Medicine along with Andre Cournand (1895–1988) for his early work in invasive cardiology.

It was Cournand, originally from Paris, who really developed modern methods for invasive studies of the heart. By inserting catheters into the heart and great vessels, he developed *cardiac catheterization* to study *hemodynamics,* which is the examination of how the heart contracts to propel blood through it. He performed his studies at Bellevue Hospital in New York City to study blood flow, pressure-volume relationships, and oxygen saturation in various parts of the heart and lungs. These methods allow a more precise understanding of the way the heart works in both acquired and congenital heart disease.

In 1960, F. Mason Sones Jr. (1918–1985), a pediatric cardiologist at the Cleveland Clinic in Ohio, accidentally injected opaque radiographic dye into the coronary artery of a patient and was able to visualize the coronary arteries. He went on to combine cardiac catheterization with coronary angiography and high-speed X-ray cinematography to visualize the coronary arteries. It was thus possible to actually see blockages within the coronary arteries. By localizing the blockages beforehand, it was possible to perform interventions such as bypass surgery and coronary angioplasty to relieve these blockages.

INTERVENTIONAL CARDIOLOGY AND CARDIAC SURGERY

Blockages in coronary arteries are the main reason for heart attacks. Now that such blockages can be actually seen and localized on moving image X-rays called *angiograms*, surgeons use veins harvested from the legs to bypass the blockages and provide blood to the heart muscle.

In the 1960s, Michael DeBakey (1908–2008) and David Sabiston (1924–2009) separately performed what is known today as *coronary artery bypass surgery* (CABG). However, it was René Favoloro (1923–2000), an Argentinean-born surgeon, who popularized CABG as the standard treatment for intractable angina. He accumulated considerable experience by repeatedly performing saphenous vein coronary bypass surgery at the Cleveland Clinic. Today, over 650,000 bypass operations are done in the United States each year. Favoloro returned to Argentina and tragically committed suicide by shooting himself in the heart during a fit of prolonged depression.

Also in 1967, Christiaan Barnard (1922–2001), a surgeon in South Africa, transplanted the first human heart from Denise Darvall into Louis Washkansky. Washkansky lived for 18 days before he died of pneumonia. Darvall was in a motor vehicle accident in Capetown and was brain damaged. Barnard injected potassium into Darvall's heart to paralyze it after obtaining permission from the parents. He then removed the heart and transplanted it. The ethical implications of removing the heart from a brain-damaged person for transplantation is a matter of debate even today. A few days later, Adrian Kantrowitz (1918–2008), in New York City, transplanted a heart from a brain-dead baby to another baby. The baby survived only six hours. Since then, thousands of successful heart transplants have been completed.

Ten years after these two seminal events in cardiac surgery, Andreas Gruentzig (1939–1985), a German radiologist, put a catheter with an inflatable balloon into a coronary artery. By applying hydrostatic pressure to inflate the balloon, he flattened plaque in a coronary artery, thus opening the artery up to increase blood flow. This procedure, called interventional cardiology or *angioplasty*, is used to relieve angina (chest pain from blocked arteries) and to prevent progression in the early stages of a heart attack.

More recently, wire mesh stents have been developed and deployed to prop the artery open. This procedure, called *stenting*, is done over a million times in the United States each year. However, these stents would clog up at a high rate due to the formation of fibrous tissue that blocked blood flow. The discovery of an antifungal agent from the soil in Easter Island called *sirolimus* (rapamycin) provided the next step in stent technology. Sirolimus was originally used to prevent rejection of organ transplants as it suppresses the immune system. This drug was also used to coat coronary stents as it retards the growth of fibrous tissue inside stents that may block the artery again. The agent elutes over a long period of time and keeps the stent open long after implantation.

Cardiac surgery has been made possible by several inventions. When the heart is being operated on, it needs to be deliberately stopped, but needs to be restarted reliably. The invention of the DC defibrillator made it possible to deliberately fibrillate the heart to operate on it, and then to restart it at the end of the operation. An infusion of a cold fluid solution can also stop the heart (*cold cardioplegia*) so that it becomes quiescent. The surgeon first places the patient on a heart-lung bypass machine to provide artificial circulation. This machine was invented by John Heysham Gibbon (1903–1973), in Philadelphia, and allows an operation to go on for several hours as needed. Then, quite deliberately, the surgeon induces VF or causes cessation of all cardiac activity (asystole) using chemical means. After surgery, defibrillation is performed or the heart is rewarmed to restore normal beating, and the patient is then taken off the heart-lung machine. Thus, several inventions over the last 100 years have come together to allow surgery to be performed safely today.

Artificial heart valves were invented by various physicians as new materials that could withstand the constant and energetic pumping of the heart were developed. The early valves were placed in the aorta by Charles Hufnagel in 1952, and later within the heart itself by Dwight Harken (in 1960) and Albert Starr and M. E. Edwards (in 1961). Concomitantly, other surgical procedures, inventions, and devices were fashioned to correct congenital heart diseases. Several inventions used together allow cardiac surgeons today to do coronary bypass surgery, replace valves, and repair holes in the heart.

In the last two decades, new approaches to surgery include minimally invasive surgery with video guidance. This method is used for coronary bypass surgery and valve repair and replacement. In addition, robotically assisted surgery is becoming more common. This method allows surgery to be done more precisely with fine adjustments to surgical technique. It also allows remote guidance for surgery if a surgeon is not immediately available on the scene using telemetry of video images.

OTHER IMPORTANT DISCOVERIES

The advent of computers and new imaging modalities has allowed the heart to be seen while in motion using ultrasound, magnetic resonance imaging, and computed tomography scanning. These methods allow the heart to be examined in great detail using noninvasive tests. Valve disorders, heart muscle abnormalities, and tumors can be seen easily in the heart through the intact chest with astounding clarity. A diagnosis can be made without opening the chest and with a high degree of accuracy to allow specific treatment options.

In the 1970s, the use of radioactive isotopes to tag blood cells showed areas in the heart to which blood was not flowing normally. A special digital camera can read the radioactive distribution of the isotope. Application of this method during an exercise stress test allows a diagnosis to be made of coronary artery disease. These technologies, often coupled with rapid computerized processing, have taken medical imaging to a new level, and well beyond what can be seen with X-rays alone.

Biochemistry and microbiology provided new diagnostic tools when the fields of chemistry and bacteriology exploded in a burst of activity in the 19th and 20th centuries. The germ theory for disease was advanced by Rudolf Virchow (1821–1902), Louis Pasteur (1822–1895), and Robert Koch (1843–1910). Developments in the 20th century led to the treatment of bacterial infections of the heart and other organs with antibiotics.

The introduction of surgical anesthesia by Crawford Long (1815–1878) in 1842 and W.T.G. Morton (1818–1868) in 1846 in the United States led to the development of safer methods for putting people to sleep and waking them up again. This development allowed the performance of prolonged and complex operations on the heart with a high degree of safety. Additionally, the discovery of blood types by Karl Landsteiner (1868–1943) in 1900 allowed blood transfusions to be done safely. This important discovery also allowed complex types of surgery to be performed directly on the heart with increasing levels of safety. Large amounts of blood may be lost during cardiac surgery, and the availability of blood is important if the patient is to survive the operation.

SUMMARY

The function of the heart has been a subject of study for over 2,000 years. However, for 1,600 of these 2,000 years, scientific study was stymied by mysticism and superstition. Moreover, the beating heart is very difficult to study as it cannot be stilled to examine it while the subject is alive.

The cumulative discoveries made over the last 400 years have been especially important in the understanding of how the heart functions and how to treat heart disease. Most of the early developments in understanding of the function of the heart and its diseases in the modern era started in Europe. However, in the last few decades, much of the research and innovation have increasingly occurred in the United States. In part this is due to the very large cost of technology needed not only to do research but also to treat patients in sufficient numbers to gather enough data.

The direction in which research is headed today suggests that studying the human genome may be useful in diagnosing heart diseases early in life. This approach may also provide treatment options directed at correcting problems at the level of the gene rather than after the disease is established.

2

Structure and Function of the Heart and Circulatory System

The heart is a supple hollow muscular organ that is constantly in motion and capable of spontaneous contraction, with an inbuilt electrical system that makes it beat normally at 60–70 beats per minute. It is the central part of the circulatory system, and the component parts of the heart are shown in Figure 2.1.

Though it weighs less than a pound, the heart is remarkably durable and forms the center of the *circulatory system*. About the size of a clenched fist, the heart in a man weighs about 12 ounces, and in a woman, only about 10 ounces. Despite its small size relative to a person's weight, it has to pump blood throughout the body and has to adapt constantly to changing states, increasing its rate and force of pumping during emotional stress and exercise and decreasing them during rest and sleep. It has to pump blood for a lifetime that, in some cases, could last over 100 years.

The heart is located slightly to the left of the midline in the chest, just behind the breastbone, so that it is protected from injury. It is essentially an electromechanical pump that has only one purpose—to pump blood that delivers oxygen and nutrients to the rest of the body. A healthy heart beats about 60–70 times a minute (somewhat faster in a child), or about 100,000 times a day. Every minute,

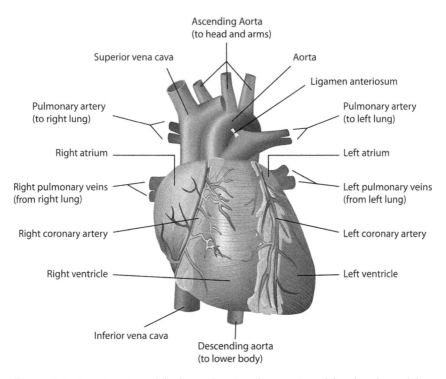

Ascending Aorta
(to head and arms)

Superior vena cava

Aorta

Ligamen anteriosum

Pulmonary artery
(to right lung)

Pulmonary artery
(to left lung)

Right atrium

Left atrium

Right pulmonary veins
(from right lung)

Left pulmonary veins
(from left lung)

Right coronary artery

Left coronary artery

Right ventricle

Left ventricle

Inferior vena cava

Descending aorta
(to lower body)

Figure 2.1 Anterior view of the heart showing the exterior of the chambers of the heart, the great vessels, and the coronary arteries. © Peterjunaidy/Dreamstime.com.

it pumps about five quarts (a little less than five liters) of blood, which comes to about 1,900 gallons (7,200 liters) each day.

The *circulatory system* is comprised of the heart, the great vessels, arteries, arterioles, veins, venules, capillaries, lymph vessels, and lymph glands. The entire circulation in an adult human is shown schematically in Figure 2.2 with the heart at its center and the arteries and veins radiating away from it or toward it. It can be seen in the diagram that the arteries and the veins track one another in very similar pathways.

If all the arteries, arterioles, veins, and capillaries that carry blood were connected end-to-end, there would be 60,000 miles of blood vessels, which is long enough to encircle the globe twice over. The main arterial trunk that springs from the heart is called the aorta. This vessel gives off arteries that subdivide into smaller arteries and then into arterioles. Arterioles divide repeatedly into smaller branches to form capillaries. The capillaries are the vessels in direct contact with cells, and it is through them that oxygen and nutrients diffuse into the cells. The capillaries reunite to form venules and these vessels unite to form veins. Veins

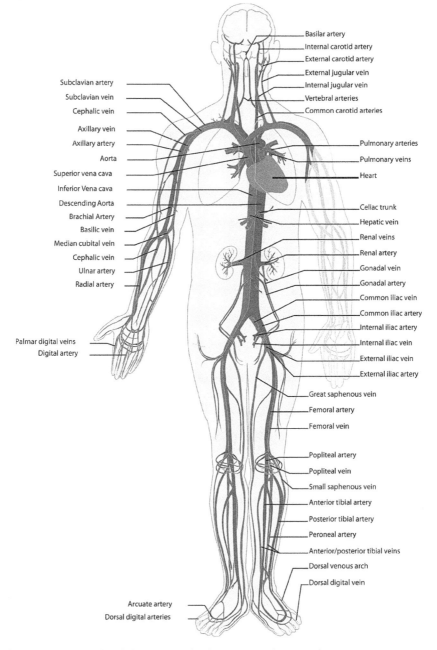

Figure 2.2 Simplified diagram of the human circulation. The major arteries are shown in dark gray and the veins are shaded in light gray. Graphic by Mariana Ruiz Villarreal.

come together to form larger veins that terminate in the vena cavae, which lead to the heart to return blood to this organ.

FUNCTIONS OF THE CIRCULATORY SYSTEM

The function of the circulation is to supply the body with oxygen and nutrition, to remove carbon dioxide, and to collect waste materials and bring them to the kidneys. The blood also serves to transport hormones and other chemically active substances to the rest of the body, from their original sources of production in various organs. These chemical substances are necessary for growth and the normal functioning of the body.

The best-known function of the lungs is *gaseous exchange*, which is the process when the lungs oxygenate blood and simultaneously remove carbon dioxide. Oxygen is vital for many cellular functions; and without oxygen, cells will deteriorate and eventually die. Organs such as the brain and heart consume very high levels of oxygen, while others, such as the gut, require less oxygen. One of the functions of the circulatory system is to channel blood to organs that require high amounts of oxygen-carrying blood while reducing blood flow to others that require less oxygen. For example, during high levels of physical activity, the muscles need more oxygen and nutrients. Therefore, the blood flow to the large muscles must increase to allow them to work faster and harder. This means that the heart has to work harder to deliver more blood to these muscles. Also, blood vessels need to dilate, or open up, to allow greater blood flow.

Regulation of the circulatory system is achieved through a part of the central nervous system called the *autonomic nervous system*. The heart and blood vessels are richly supplied by nerves from the autonomic nervous system (ANS). The circulatory system is extremely responsive to inputs from the brain through the ANS. The ANS is made up of two components: the *sympathetic* and *parasympathetic* systems. The sympathetic nervous system (SNS) increases heart rate and the force of the heart's pumping action, and causes constriction of blood vessels. The parasympathetic nervous system (PSNS) does the very opposite. Thus, the ANS has a "push-pull" effect on the actions of the heart and the circulation of blood. By the actions of the ANS, heart rate, cardiac output of blood, and blood flow through the arteries can be altered or adjusted, depending on physical needs during exercise, severe psychological stress, sleep, and so forth.

The sympathetic nervous system is responsible for stimulating the heart to increase the heart rate and blood pressure during exercise. This is important as oxygen and nutritional requirements increase during exercise, and blood supply to muscles has to be increased to meet this demand. The SNS also stimulates the release of adrenaline by the adrenal glands. Adrenaline is carried by the blood throughout the circulatory system to increase heart rate and blood pressure by stimulating arterioles to contract. During sleep, the parasympathetic nervous system slows down the heart and this reduces oxygen consumption. Overactivity of the PSNS can cause severe slowing of the heart rate, or lowering of the blood pressure, leading to dizziness and fainting.

The ANS also has a role in temperature regulation via the circulation. In cold weather, the ANS regulates blood flow to the skin by constricting peripheral blood vessels, thereby reducing heat loss. Thus, the relationship between the two components of the ANS and the circulatory system is very close and the two branches of the ANS oppose one another.

In old age, and with certain diseases, such as diabetes, the nerves of the ANS become less responsive or they actually become damaged. These conditions lead to imbalances in blood pressure, heart rate, and the ability to regulate blood flow to various organs. When this occurs, fine-tuning of the circulatory system by the ANS is lost, resulting in symptoms such as weakness, dizziness, and fainting. The ability to exercise is also impaired by age and diabetes, when the heart and blood vessels have lost their ability to function normally under physical stress.

ARCHITECTURE OF THE HEART

The normal human heart, like all mammalian hearts, is divided internally into four sections, or chambers. If you imagine the heart as a four-roomed house, there would be two rooms upstairs, called *atria* (singular: *atrium*), and two rooms downstairs, the *ventricles*. The walls that separate the chambers are called *septa* (singular: *septum*). Each of the upstairs chambers is connected to the downstairs chambers by trapdoor-like valves. The *tricuspid valve* lies between the right atrium and the right ventricle. The *mitral valve* lets blood flow from the left atrium into the left ventricle.

Blood vessels that conduct blood away from the heart are called *arteries*, while blood vessels that return blood to the heart are called *veins*. The outflow of blood from the left ventricle is ejected through the aortic valve into the aorta. The output from the right ventricle is pumped into the pulmonary artery through the pulmonary valve. The aorta and the pulmonary artery are also called the *great vessels*. The aorta distributes oxygenated, or "red," blood to the whole body. The pulmonary artery carries deoxygenated, or "blue," blood to the lungs to pick up oxygen. Since each side of the heart consists of one atrium and one ventricle, it is conventional to speak of the heart as having two functional sides: the *left heart* and the *right heart*. Though the two sides of the heart are attached to one another, their physiological behavior is different, and disease conditions may affect predominantly one side and not the other.

The major components are the following interconnected structures:

Atria—the two upper chambers
Ventricles—the two lower chambers
Valves—four in number (aortic, pulmonic, mitral, and tricuspid)
Coronary arteries—the two major vessels that feed the heart with blood
The great vessels and the peripheral circulation—the aorta, pulmonary artery, and their respective branches
Conduction system—the electrical cable system that wires the heart
Pericardium—the thin translucent covering over the heart

The Atria

The atria (the upper rooms of the heart) are chambers for holding blood and are very thin-walled. They have a weak pumping action and can squeeze blood into the ventricles below them. The atria are connected to the ventricles by the mitral and tricuspid valves. The atria are essentially receiving chambers. The right atrium receives deoxygenated blood from the superior vena cava and the inferior vena cava. The left atrium receives oxygenated blood from the lungs through the pulmonary veins.

Embedded in the wall of the right atrium is a small bundle of electrically active cells called the *sinoatrial (SA) node*. This is the normal and natural pacemaker that fires regularly and drives the heart at a resting rate of 60–70 beats per minute, but it can fire at a more rapid rate, if necessary. It is connected to the electrical conduction of the heart to keep the beating regular. With age, the SA node progressively slows down and sometimes stops firing completely, leading to a condition called *asystole* when there is no heartbeat.

The Ventricles

The lower chambers, or ventricles, are the pumping chambers of the heart, and they have thicker walls than the atria. The left ventricle is thicker than the right ventricle and is more powerful in its pumping action.

The ventricular muscle is made up of a special kind of muscle called *unstriated muscle*. It is different from skeletal, or *striated*, muscle in that it has the ability to start contracting on its own if there is no stimulation from the normal cardiac pacemaker. However, its own intrinsic beat is only about 20–40 beats per minute, while the normal resting heartbeat is about 60–80 beats per minute. In children the resting rate is higher and may be 100 or 110 beats per minute. The ventricular muscle is made up of three sections: the *epicardium*, the *myocardium*, and the *endocardium*.

The *epicardium* is thin and forms the outermost layer of the heart. The thick muscular middle layer that contracts forcefully is the *myocardium*. The innermost thin layer that lines the inner walls of the ventricles is the *endocardium*. The blood supply to the heart muscle is richest in the outer layer closest to the coronary arteries. When a myocardial infarction occurs, it may involve only the outermost layers of the heart, only the innermost layers, or the entire thickness of the muscle.

When the ventricles contract, blood is squeezed out of the heart; this action is called *systole* (*systo-lee*). There is always some blood still left in the left ventricle at the end of systole, and the residual amount of blood is called the *end-systolic volume (ESV)*. This volume left in each ventricle is about 50 milliliters in a normal 70-kilogram man. When the ventricles relax after each beat to fill with blood, this period of time is called *diastole* (*diasto-lee*). When the ventricles are full of blood, the volume of blood is called the *end-diastolic volume (EDV)*, which is usually about 120 milliliters in the each ventricle.

The difference between the EDV and the ESV is called the *stroke volume (SV)*. This is the volume of blood ejected into the aorta or pulmonary artery with every heartbeat. This relationship can be expressed by the following equation:

$$EDV - ESV = SV$$

Though the volumes are the same for both ventricles, by convention, only the left ventricular volumes are used as an overall measure of cardiac function. Using the end-diastolic and end-systolic values given above, the stroke volume of the left ventricle is 70 milliliters in a 70-kilogram man. The stroke volume divided by the end-diastolic volume is called the *ejection fraction (EF)* of the left ventricle, which is expressed as a percentage as follows:

$$\frac{SV}{EDV} \times 100 = \text{Ejection fraction (\%)}$$

Again, using the numbers above, we can calculate the ejection fraction for the left ventricle as follows:

$$\frac{70}{120} \times 100 = 58\%$$

The normal left ventricular ejection fraction lies in the range of 55–70 percent in the adult. Ejection fraction can be measured during cardiac catheterization by the injection of dye into the left ventricle to outline it radiographically on an X-ray movie film while it is contracting, and then calculating the difference between the end of diastole and the end of systole. The same process can also be applied by echocardiography, or by radionuclide scanning, both of which will outline the left ventricle while it is pumping.

When the left ventricle is damaged during myocardial infarction or by cardiomyopathy, the EF decreases. If the EF decreases to below 35 percent, there is a higher risk of congestive heart failure. People can live with an EF as low as 15 percent, though they cannot exert themselves very much. The EF is also important as the risk of sudden cardiac death is increased with a decline in EF to 35 percent or less. Long-term survival after a myocardial infarction is more likely when the EF is relatively well preserved after recovery and is well above 35 percent.

The heart alternates between systole and diastole, beating about 60–70 times a minute at rest in an adult. If we multiply the stroke volume by the heart rate (HR), we will get a measure of the amount of blood pumped out of the heart per minute. The resulting number is called the cardiac output (CO). This relationship is mathematically represented as:

$$HR \times SV = CO \text{ (liters/minute)}$$

Since the normal heart rate is about 70 beats per minute and the stroke volume is about 70 milliliters (or 0.07 liters), the cardiac output in an adult can be calculated as below:

$$70 \times 0.07 = 4.9 \text{ (liters/minute)}$$

As shown in the equation above, the normal cardiac output in an adult is about 5 liters per minute, but this value can increase or decrease depending on the circumstances. During exercise or excitement, adrenaline and sympathetic nerve stimulation make the heart beat faster, and rates as high as 220 beats may result. The ejection fraction also increases with exercise and excitement as the heart contracts more powerfully, ejecting more blood. Therefore, if the heart contracts more vigorously during exercise and stroke volume increases to 90 milliliters with each heartbeat, and the heart rate increases to 100 per minute, the cardiac output will almost double to 9 liters per minute. The increases in contractile force and heart rate are necessary to increase blood flow, which provides more oxygen to the muscles during exercise or to get ready for the *fight or flight* response during real or anticipated danger.

Sometimes, runaway rhythms occur that may result from excessive adrenaline, or from some disorder of the conduction system itself. If the heart rate is too rapid (e.g., 250 beats per minute), there is very little time between beats for the heart to fill up with enough blood during diastole. When this happens, the reduced filling time of the heart and very rapid rate actually results in a decrease in cardiac output due to a decline in the heart's mechanical efficiency. This situation results in a decrease in blood pressure and the person may become dizzy and even pass out.

The heart is therefore a dynamic organ that is extremely responsive to physiological and psychological changes. It can adapt itself to a wide variety of conditions by both internal autoregulation and by regulation of heart rate and contractility through the autonomic nervous system.

The Heart Valves

Valves are structures that allow one-way flow of gases or fluids. There are four main valves in the human heart. The *mitral* and *tricuspid* valves sit between the atria and the ventricles. The *aortic* and *pulmonic valves* guard the exit from the ventricles into the aorta and the pulmonary artery respectively. As seen in Figure 2.3, the pulmonic valve is at the root of the pulmonary artery and the aortic valve is partially hidden by the ascending part of the same artery.

At the beginning of systole, the mitral and tricuspid valves close to prevent backwash of blood into the atria from which blood has just been emptied. During systole, the aortic and pulmonic valves open and allow blood to exit the ventricles and enter the lung circulation and the systemic circulation. The reverse occurs during diastole, where the mitral and tricuspid valves open and let blood enter the ventricles that the aortic and pulmonic valves close. The ventricles fill with blood during diastole, and the cycle of the valves opening and closing is then repeated.

Heart valves are made up of thin translucent tissue that looks like cellophane. Each valve is mounted on a ring that is somewhat elastic. Each valve has either two or three leaflets, each of which is called a cusp. The mitral valve is bicuspid, meaning there are two cusps. The aortic, pulmonic, and tricuspid valves have three cusps. One of the most common congenital abnormalities is when the aortic valve has only two cusps, instead of three. Though the valve functions normally, it is likely to become calcified and narrowed earlier than normal three-cusp valves.˙

Down in the ventricles, there are string-like cords (*chordae tendinae*) that are attached to the underside of the valves, like the ropes that are attached to a sail. These cords are in turn attached to small muscular posts, which are called *papillary muscles*. The chordae tendinae hold the valve leaflets together and prevent

Internal anatomy of the heart

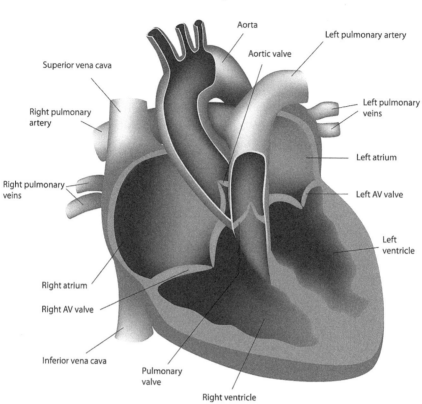

Aorta

Left pulmonary artery

Aortic valve

Superior vena cava

Left pulmonary veins

Right pulmonary artery

Left atrium

Right pulmonary veins

Left AV valve

Left ventricle

Right atrium

Right AV valve

Inferior vena cava

Pulmonary valve

Right ventricle

Figure 2.3 Internal anatomy of the heart. Cutaway diagram showing the heart and its four chambers. The pulmonary artery arises from the right ventricle and the pulmonary valve is at its base. Underneath, the aorta arises from the left ventricle and part of the aortic valve can be seen behind the pulmonary artery. The right AV (atrioventricular) valve is the tricuspid valve and the left AV valve is the mitral valve (right and left designations refer to the person's right and left sides). © Alila07/Dreamstime.com.

them from inverting or blowing out into the atria above them when the ventricles power up and contract. As pressure mounts in the ventricles during systole, the valves billow upward and snap shut. If the chordae do not hold them down, they will be blown into the atria and blood will leak back into the atria. In some disease states that destroy the chordae, this is exactly what happens, thus allowing for the blowback of blood.

In certain disease conditions, valves can be damaged and narrowed, resulting in decreased blood flow. This condition is called *stenosis*, or the narrowing of the valvular orifice. If the valves do not close properly, backward leakage of blood occurs, and this is called *valvular insufficiency* or *regurgitation*. Aging of the valves and rheumatic fever can cause valvular stenosis. Rheumatic fever can also cause valvular regurgitation. Sometimes, stenosis and regurgitation can coexist in the same valve. In such cases, the valve not only impedes forward flow, but also leaks, allowing a backflow of blood that makes the condition worse.

Problems with partial blockage or leakage of the valves lead to inefficient pumping, as would be the case with any pump. This reduces the mechanical capability of the heart to pump blood, especially if either condition is severe, and the valve needs to be repaired or replaced as explained in chapters 4 and 10. Valves are necessary for the proper functioning of the heart, and their normal action allows maximization of efficiency in maintaining the steady forward flow of blood.

The Coronary Arteries

The coronary arteries get their name from the Latin word *corona* (meaning "crown") because they fully encircle the heart in the groove between the atria on top and the ventricles below. There are two main arteries, the left coronary artery and the right coronary artery. Both coronary arteries come off the root of the aorta just as it emerges from the left ventricle (Figure 2.1).

The left coronary artery (LCA) is generally the larger artery and is called the dominant artery. This artery begins as the left main coronary artery (LMCA), which is short, and it quickly divides into two parts soon after it emerges from the aorta. One branch runs down the front of the heart and is called the left anterior descending artery (LAD) and the other branch, called the diagonal artery, runs off to the side of the left ventricle. The LCA feeds mostly the left ventricle and the anterior two-thirds of the interventricular septum. Therefore, blockage of the LMCA can be very serious as the left ventricle will be massively damaged. Blockage of the LAD is also serious as it can result in damage to the front of the heart as this is mainly made up of the left ventricle. Damage to the conduction system of the heart, which is supplied by this artery, is also serious as complete heart block can occur and the patient may die, even if a pacemaker is inserted to control heart rate.

The right coronary is usually smaller and supplies the right ventricle and the back of the interventricular septum. Blockage of this artery can cause angina and myocardial infarction. However, the damage caused is less extensive than that with blockages of the left coronary system as the amount of muscle fed by this artery is small. Though blockage of this artery can also cause electrical heart block, it is generally relatively benign and reversible. Diseases affecting the coronary arteries are described later, along with the consequences of such conditions. Interventional medical and surgical treatments to correct coronary blockages will also be described in Chapters 3 and 10.

The Great Vessels and the Peripheral Circulation

The term *great vessels* is applied to the two main arteries that emerge from the ventricles. The aorta emerges from the left ventricle and carries oxygenated blood to the entire body. The pulmonary artery exits from the right ventricle and carries venous blood to the lungs to be oxygenated. Though not strictly part of the heart, the great vessels are closely attached to the heart. Some cardiac abnormalities, such as Tetralogy of Fallot and transposition of the great vessels affect not only the heart, but also the great vessels. Conversely, diseases of the root of the aorta, such as dissection, can track backward into the root of the aorta and affect the coronary arteries. In treating these conditions, the heart and great vessels need to be considered as one unit.

The great vessels give off major branches that divide into smaller arteries, which in turn divide into even smaller arterioles. All of these vessels have three concentric layers. The outermost layer is the *adventitia*, the middle layer is the *media*, and the innermost layer is the *intima*. The outermost layer is mostly connective tissue and serves to hold the inner layers in place. The middle layer is made up of smooth muscle cells and elastic tissue. The larger arteries, such as the aorta and its larger branches, have thick walls and a great deal of elastic tissue in the middle layer that can withstand the pressure generated by the heart. The inner layer is the *intima*, which is made up of one layer of endothelial cells that is virtually frictionless and allows for the smooth flow of blood.

The smaller arteries and the arterioles have a slightly different structure. Their middle walls have a large amount of muscular tissue that allows contraction and expansion of the vessel. There is considerable control of this function by the sympathetic nervous system. As described earlier, during periods of exercise, the arterioles can expand to provide more blood to the muscles and organs that need it. It is the arterioles that also ultimately control what the blood pressure reading will be. If they constrict, the blood pressure will be raised; and if they expand, blood pressure decreases.

Arterioles divide into capillaries that are very small and thin-walled. It is from the capillaries that the oxygen and nutrients diffuse toward the cells that require nutrition. The capillaries reunite to form venules that merge into veins.

The veins rejoin other veins to form large vessels called the *vena cavae*, which bring blood back to the right side of the heart. This process completes the circuit of blood that travels from the left side of the heart to the right side of the heart.

The Conduction System of the Heart

Though the heart muscle is capable of beating on its own, the spontaneous rate of the ventricles (the *idioventricular rate*) is low and only around 20 40 beats per minute. The heart is really an electromechanical system, very much like a gasoline-powered car engine. An engine does not function until it is triggered by an electrical system that ignites fuel and makes the engine run. Similarly, there is an electrical system that consists of a *pacemaker* embedded in the wall of the right atrium and is connected to a system of cables that runs throughout the heart. The pacemaker is roughly analogous to an ignition system that gives off electrical sparks that ignite the fuel. The cardiac pacemaker is made of a cluster of electrically active cells that are capable of spontaneous electrical discharge sixty times or so a minute. These electrical impulses are conducted down the cables that ramify throughout the heart and fire the muscle tissue to make the atria and ventricles contract mechanically. The entire system is called the *electrical conduction system* of the heart and its components can be summarized as follows:

- The *sinoatrial node* in the upper right atrium.
- *Bachmann's Bundle*, extending from the sinoatrial node to the high left atrium.
- The *atrioventricular node* sits between the atria and the ventricles (also called *the junction*).
- The *Bundle of His* is a short stretch of cable leading from the AV node into the ventricles and divides into the bundle branches.
- The *bundle branches*, which come off the Bundle of His, have two major divisions called the *left bundle branch* and the *right bundle branch*. Each bundle is located within its respective side of the interventricular septum.
- The bundle branches branch repeatedly in the ventricular muscle into *Purkinje fibers* that innervate individual groups of myocardial cells to make them contract.

An electrical impulse originating spontaneously in the sinoatrial (SA) node depolarizes the atria, producing the P-wave on the EKG (Figure 2.4). The impulse then travels through Bachmann's Bundle to another tight clump of electrically active tissue called the *atrioventricular (AV) node* that sits in the center of the heart at the junction between the atria and ventricles. The time from initiation of the impulse to the arrival at the AV node is called the PR-interval. From the AV node the impulse travels through the Bundle of His and then into the ventricles through the bundle branches. One branch, the right bundle branch, innervates the right ventricle. The other branch, the left bundle branch, innervates the left ventricle.

The impulse then travels into the ventricles to Purkinje fibers that activate the two ventricles simultaneously, making them contract, producing the QRS-complex. The contraction of the ventricles propels blood forward out of the ventricles into the lungs and into the general circulation of the body. The ventricle then relaxes after the electrical depolarization wave that sweeps over the entire ventricular mass is concluded. The myocardial muscle then recharges itself by ionic exchange across the cell membrane. The recharging or repolarization period can be seen in Figure 2.4 as the T-wave. The U-wave that follows is Purkinje fiber repolarization.

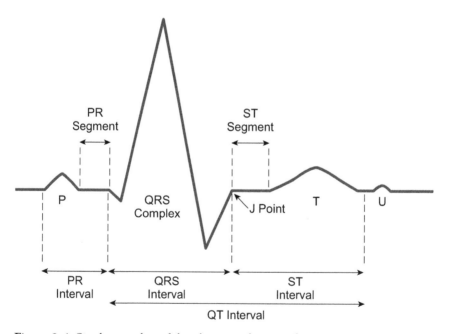

Figure 2.4 Single complex of the electrocardiogram showing waves and electrocardiographic intervals.

The sequence as summarized in Figure 2.4 is as follows:

- P-wave: Atrial depolarization (activation)
- PR-interval: Duration from onset of atrial depolarization to onset of ventricular depolarization
- QRS-interval: Duration of right and left ventricular depolarization (activation)
- ST-interval: Duration of ventricular repolarization
- ST-segment: Return to isoelectric baseline after ventricular depolarization
- QT-interval: Total duration of ventricular depolarization and repolarization
- J-point: Marks the end of the QRS-complex and the beginning of the ST-segment

We shall come back to the ST-segment and the J-point in chapter 8 in the section on exercise stress testing.

This sequential activation of the atria followed shortly thereafter by ventricular activation is repeated about 60–70 times a minute, producing a heartbeat that is felt at the wrist as a pulse. Because the SA node is richly innervated by the sympathetic nervous system during exercise or excitement, the heart rate increases, reaching up to 180–200 times a minute.

How exactly does an electrical impulse cause the heart muscle to contract? The heart is an electrical organ, much like the brain. As described, the arrival of an electrical impulse from the sinoatrial node down to the atrioventricular node and into the ventricles causes a spreading wave that completely envelops the muscular tissue. This impulse sets off a chain reaction that results in muscular contraction using glucose as the energy source and powered by adenosine triphosphate (ATP). The cell membranes of muscles contain small sodium-potassium "pumps." These pumps change the electrical charge on the surface of the cell so that there is a negative charge on the outside and a positive charge on the inside of the cell membrane. When an electrical impulse arrives down the bundle branches and permeates the ventricular muscle, they cause the electrical charge on the cell membrane surface to reverse itself suddenly. The process occurs because a massive efflux of sodium leaves the cell suddenly and potassium flows inward into the cell. This extremely rapid event is called *depolarization* of the cell membrane and it generates an *action potential*, described in chapter 1. When millions of cells in the ventricles are depolarized synchronously, the result is a strong muscular contraction that lasts only for about 80 milliseconds.

Since this electrical phenomenon occurs in all the cells of the ventricles almost simultaneously, the result is a coordinated and synchronized contraction of the entire right and left ventricular muscle mass. The entire process is called *electromechanical coupling*. The event is over extremely quickly, in less than 0.8 seconds, which is the duration of the QRS-complex. The ventricles then relax and recharge electrically by a reversal of the flow of sodium back into the cell and potassium being pumped out of the cell. The ventricles then await the next electrical impulse to come down the pike and depolarize them again.

A rhythm disturbance can occur in two ways. There may be an abnormal focus of electrical activity arising somewhere in the atria or around the AV node itself, thus capturing the heart and overtaking the normal heartbeat. This abnormal focus acts as an *ectopic pacemaker* and overcomes the function of the normal pacemaker in the SA node. These abnormal impulses can travel down the bundle branches and force the ventricles to beat at a very high rate, even at 300 times a minute or more.

The AV node has some peculiar features that distinguish it from the SA node. If the atria beat at over 300 beats a minute, the AV node acts as an electrical "gate" and blocks the impulses from getting down into the ventricles. This gating function cuts down the number of impulses that can get through. The blocking function is such that only every second, third, or fourth impulse gets through to provoke the ventricles into action. This condition is called *heart block* and should be differentiated from actual physical blockage of coronary arteries that causes myocardial infarction. If the atria beat at 300 times a minute, and if only every second beat gets through, then the ventricles will beat at 150 times a minute. This phenomenon is called 2:1 block. And if every third beat gets through, and the other two impulses are blocked, the ventricular rate is 100 beats per minute (3:1 block). An electrical "block" prevents the ventricles from beating too rapidly to be effective in pumping out blood. This kind of block is a protective device as it prevents a "runaway" rhythm that can make a person faint. However, sometimes the AV node itself creates its own mischief and can generate abnormal impulses at a high rate, making the heart beat at 200 or 300 times a minute.

A second way the ventricles may beat too rapidly is if there is an abnormal or ectopic focus in the ventricles themselves that take over the function of a pacemaker. Such a condition can occur spontaneously or arise if there is heart muscle damage (e.g., during myocardial infarction). If only one or a few abnormal beats occur, these beats are called ventricular premature beats and no great harm comes to the patient. As the heart ages, these extra beats are quite commonly seen on an EKG. However, if the beats are repetitive and sustained, this condition is called *ventricular tachycardia*. Ventricular tachycardia leads to cardiac arrest and death in some cases, as will be described later.

Sometimes, the entire ventricle goes haywire and the depolarization sequence is disrupted to such an extent that the heart's electrical activity becomes completely chaotic. This condition, called *ventricular fibrillation*, results in sudden death if it is not electrically reversed by electrical defibrillation. The evaluation of the integrity of the electrical system of the heart and the main cardiac rhythm disturbances and their treatment are described later. Treatments may include medications, pacemakers, implantable defibrillators, catheter ablation, and surgical treatments that interrupt or correct abnormalities of the electrical conduction system of the heart.

The Pericardium

The entire heart, except for the left atrium, is encased in a thin transparent sac called the pericardium. It is made up of two layers, the outer fibrous pericardium and an inner parietal layer.

Though the pericardium is not essential for life, it keeps the heart in its proper position in the chest cavity. It also serves to secure the heart as an external brace to prevent overexpansion of the heart when it fills with blood. This function probably improves the heart's pumping efficiency by constraining it in its proper shape. The pressure within the sac is below atmospheric pressure, and this probably also adds to the efficient functioning of the heart. The pericardium serves to prevent friction between the heart and the surrounding tissue, as its pumping action causes rotational torsion while it squeezes blood out of the ventricles. The pericardium also protects the heart from infections and other processes that may affect the surrounding lung tissue.

A quantity of about 15–50 cubic centimeters of clear serous fluid lubricates the space between the two layers of the pericardium. In certain diseases the amount of fluid increases considerably, and this condition is called *pericardial effusion*. Up to 1.6 liters of fluid may accumulate in some cases. If excessive fluid accumulates, the pumping action of the heart is compromised in a condition called *pericardial tamponade*. If inflammation of the pericardium occurs, the heart becomes impaired, and the condition is called *constrictive pericarditis*. These conditions may be life-threatening if left untreated as the heart is compressed by fluid and cannot pump effectively.

In disease conditions such as constrictive pericarditis, the pericardium may need to be removed. Such removal does not seem to impair functioning of the heart significantly. Similarly, during cardiac bypass surgery, the pericardium is cut into, and stripping away the pericardium does not appear to cause any long-term problems.

The Circulation of Blood

The sole purpose of the heart is to pump blood around the body and to keep it moving. The point of entry of blood into the heart from the rest of the body is the right atrium of the heart. Blood arrives at the right atrium from the rest of the body via the superior and inferior vena cavae. The superior vena cava drains blood from the head and upper part of the body, and the inferior vena cava brings in blood to the heart from the lower two-thirds of the body. From the right atrium, blood is delivered into the right ventricle through the tricuspid valve. From there it is then pumped out of the heart into the pulmonary artery coursing through the pulmonic valve. Blood then moves through the lung circulation carried by fine capillaries to tiny air sacs called *alveoli,* where the venous blood picks up oxygen. This process, called *oxygenation,* is accompanied by release of carbon dioxide from the blood into the alveoli.

Blood from the alveoli is collected by small capillaries that merge into venules and then into veins that unite and ultimately drain through the four large pulmonary veins into the left atrium. The oxygenated blood in the left atrium then practically falls through gravity into the left ventricle through the mitral valve. The newly oxygenated blood is then pumped out of the left ventricle into the aorta, through the aortic valve, and is then distributed to the rest of the body. The aorta branches out into arteries that further subdivide into arterioles and into tiny capillaries. It is the capillaries that distribute blood directly into the tissues that consume oxygen and nutrients that keep the capillaries alive.

After it courses throughout the body, when oxygen and nutrients have been extracted from it, the depleted blood is channeled by capillaries that join to form venules. Veins are formed by the confluence of venules, and blood returns to the right atrium via the superior vena cava and the inferior vena cava.

Therefore, the circulatory system is made up of two interlocking and physically separate loops. One loop involves the right side of the heart containing depleted dark venous blood, and the other involves the left side of the heart containing red oxygen-rich blood. In a normal heart, these loops are kept completely separate, and mixing of the *deoxygenated* (blue) blood and the *oxygenated* (red) blood does not normally occur. However, as we will see later, when there are congenital abnormalities of the heart (e.g., holes in the heart), blood crosses over from one side of the heart to the other.

There is another difference between the two sides: the left heart is a *high-pressure system* that packs considerable force. This is because it has to pump blood to the entire body, which puts considerable physical stress on the left heart. It also has to work against relatively high blood pressure in the aorta, so the left ventricle has to be thicker and more powerful than the right ventricle. The right side is a *low-pressure system,* as it has to pump blood only to the lungs, which is basically a honeycomb of air sacs that offers little resistance to blood flow. Therefore, the right ventricle is thin-walled and not as well-powered as the left.

Due to the difference in the pressures of the left heart system and the right heart system, blood will flow from the left side to the right side if there is a hole in the heart in some forms of congenital heart disease, as we shall see in chapter 7. In the case of *atrial septal defect*, blood flows from the left atrium to the right atrium through a hole in the atrial septum. In the case of a hole in the ventricular septum, blood flows from the high-pressure left ventricle to the low-pressure right ventricle. This abnormal situation results in *volume overload* of the right heart due to the fact that the right side now has to deal with up to twice the volume of blood. Obviously, this is not a good situation, and it leads to *congestive heart failure*, where the heart simply cannot pump effectively due to the overload of blood flowing through it.

The normal circulation of blood through the heart and its chambers to the rest of the body is summarized quantitatively in Table 2.1. The table shows the mechanical aspects of cardiac action and how the heart powers the movement of blood through itself and throughout the rest of the body. The mathematical relationships between pressure, volume, and flow are collectively called *hemodynamics*, which literally means "blood movement," or movement of the blood.

Hemodynamic function of the heart is an important part of cardiac physiology and when it is disordered by loss of blood volume or malfunction of the heart, serious consequences occur that can result in the death of the person. The objective of treatment in many disorders of the heart, such as congestive heart failure, is to restore the normal hemodynamics of the heart by using drugs or by surgical means. Under normal conditions, the heart functions marvelously and sustains life for a very long period of time.

Table 2.1 The heart and circulation in an adult male human

Heart weight (oz)	12
Number of chambers	4
Number of valves	4
Number of coronary arteries	2
Miles of blood vessels	60,000
Volume of blood (liters)	5
Resting heart rate (beats/min)	70
Stroke volume (cc)	70
Ejection fraction (%)	60
Cardiac output (liters/min)	5
Peak systolic blood pressure (mmHg)	120
Diastolic pressure (mmHg)	80
End-diastolic volume (cc)	120
End-systolic volume (cc)	50

SUMMARY

The cardiovascular system is responsible for providing a delivery mechanism for blood that nourishes the entire body. It delivers oxygen, nutrients, hormones, and blood cells that protect the body from infection to all organs in the body. The heart, the centerpiece of the circulatory system, is a remarkably stout organ that pumps blood for a lifetime without resting. It is essentially an electromechanical organ consisting of a pump that is electrically wired to keep it beating in response to physiological demands. It has a remarkable capacity to slow down during rest and sleep, and to increase its force and rate of pumping when the person exercises or becomes excited.

The healthy heart can last a lifetime of a 100 years or more, though a more typical lifespan is about 60 to 80 years in the West. In succeeding chapters, we will describe the diseases that can affect the heart's normal functioning and how death may occur from these conditions if they are not properly treated.

3

Disorders of Coronary Circulation

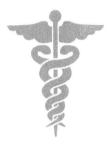

Case Study

JB was a tall, lanky, 67-year-old retired metal foundry worker who felt a burning sensation, like a "blowtorch," in his chest when he exerted himself. Sometimes, the discomfort came on when he was emotionally upset. His wife died about six months before I saw him. He was very depressed over her death and he missed her very much. A resting electrocardiogram (EKG) was normal, but a stress test was markedly abnormal for changes of ischemia in the anterior and inferior walls of the heart. The pumping action of his heart was normal with no evidence of previous damage. A coronary angiogram showed severe blockages in three arteries, and coronary bypass surgery was done the following week. He did very well for two years with no angina, but he remained deeply depressed. Due to palpitations and dizziness, a Holter tape monitor was applied to record his EKG in order to assess his cardiac rhythm. While it was still in place, his daughter found him dead in bed the next morning. She returned the Holter monitor a few days later and analysis of the EKG recording showed ventricular fibrillation as the cause of death. On further discussion with his daughter, it was discovered that the anniversary of his wife's death was two days before his death, and his wedding anniversary was the day following his death.

Diseases of the heart are the single greatest cause of death, disease, and disability in the United States and the Western world. Heart disease accounts for 40 percent of deaths in the United States and far exceeds cancer, stroke, and accidents, as shown in Table 3.1.

Table 3.1 Causes of death in the United States (2006)

Heart diseases	631,636
Cancers	559,888
Strokes	137,119
Lung diseases	124,583
Accidents	121,599
Diabetes	72,449

Most of the cardiac deaths are due to coronary artery disease (CAD), and totaled 595,444 by 2010. Strokes accounted for 129,180 deaths for a total of 724,624 for all cardiovascular deaths counted as one entity.

In comparison, there were 573,855 deaths from cancer by 2010. In the last decade there were 40,820 deaths from breast cancer and 28,372 from prostate cancer approximately each year, which is far less than those from heart disease. Deaths from HIV/AIDS in the United States and its five dependent territories numbered 17,374 annually. Numbers for Western European countries are approximately similar in terms of the proportion of deaths from CAD compared to other causes. Since death from CAD is the leading cause of mortality in the West, it is a very large part of the economic burden in both the United States and Europe.

In rapidly developing countries like India, China, Brazil, and Argentina, higher standards of living, richer foods, and the stress of modern life are leading to an increase in death rates from heart disease. In years to come, CAD will replace infectious disease and malnutrition as the leading cause of death and disease in these countries, as it has in the Western world. This disease strikes men and women in the prime of life and exacts a large toll on the workforce. Besides the need to understand and treat heart disease for its own sake, the economic implications of this disease on a nation are significant and a demographic dividend can be gained if deaths from cardiovascular disease can be successfully contained.

ORIGINS OF CAD

CAD is the most common type of heart disease affecting almost 13 million people in the United States, causing death and disability due to *ventricular arrhythmias* (serious disorders of the heartbeat), *angina pectoris* (chest pains due to lack of blood supply to the heart), and *myocardial infarction* (heart muscle damage).

As described in chapter 1, the heart has two main coronary arteries that carry oxygen-rich blood to heart muscle. These vessels may become blocked in two ways. First, there may be blockages that develop gradually with age by plaque buildup, or by damage from various disease processes that cause CAD. Second, a normal artery may develop coronary spasm, choking off blood supply. In the latter case, there is no true blockage, but the vessel constricts due to the smooth muscle in the wall contracting and narrowing the diameter of the artery. The throttling of blood supply is temporary, but this may lead to chest pain and cause heart damage in some people. It is possible for spasm to occur on top of a partially blocked artery, making it much worse. This condition is known as *variant angina*, or Prinzmetal's angina (named for Myron Prinzmetal [1908–1987], who first described this condition). Various other unusual causes of CAD include cocaine and recreational drug use, and rheumatic diseases such as rheumatoid arthritis and polyarteritis nodosa. These toxins and disease processes damage the arterial walls, leading to obstructions that cause blood flow problems.

Arteries are made up of three concentric layers. The outer *adventitial layer* is made up of tough connective tissue that prevents overexpansion of the artery due to the high pressures within it. The middle layer, or *media,* is made of smooth muscle and elastic fibers that allow for contraction and expansion of the vessel diameter. The very thin inner layer, or *intimal layer,* has a very smooth surface called the *endothelium,* along which blood and blood cells can glide with minimal friction and without clotting. The left image in Figure 3.1 shows the three layers of a normal artery in cutaway section.

The endothelium develops plaque buildup over the years because of wear and tear and due to the deposition of cholesterol and other substances. As the person ages, a gritty or chalky substance made up of these materials begins to accumulate on the inner intimal layer so that the surface looks like it is lined with popcorn, as shown in the right-hand image in Figure 3.1. The lining may also become damaged by the stress of blood flowing at high pressures over many years. *Risk factors* such as high blood pressure, high levels of cholesterol, and smoking promote the development of plaque, as discussed in Chapter 12. When plaque builds up in the arteries, the condition is called *atherosclerosis,* and this is the basis for most CAD. Other terms for CAD are coronary heart disease and ischemic heart disease.

Plaque is made up of fat, cholesterol, calcium, and other substances found in the blood. There are two kinds of plaque: *hard plaque* and *soft plaque*. Hard plaques are solid, contain calcium, and are quite stable, meaning that they do not break open. Soft plaques are covered with a soft fibrous cap and are more likely to be vulnerable to bursting open under physical stress. It is thought that the plaque ruptures suddenly when it becomes unstable, thereby releasing its contents. Such

ATHEROSCLEROSIS

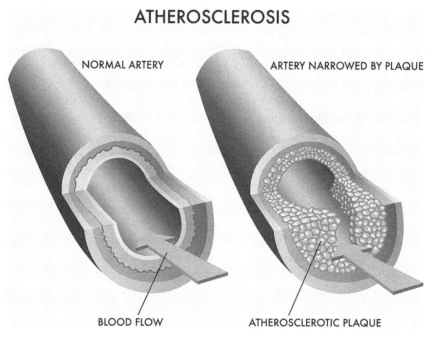

Figure 3.1 Normal structure of an artery and development of atherosclerosis. Cutaway of an artery showing three layers in the left panel: the outer layer (adventitia), the middle layer (media), and the inner layer (intima). The right panel shows the intima filled with popcorn-like plaque partially obstructing the lumen of the artery. © Rob3000/Dreamstime.com.

rupture can occur spontaneously, during exertion or during emotional stress, or during sudden rises in blood pressure. The rough surface of the ruptured plaque acts as a platform for a blood clot to form when platelets and red and white blood cells clump together. The clot forms rapidly and quickly turns a partial blockage into a complete, 100 percent, blockage. Such a complete blockage totally chokes off blood to the heart muscle supplied by this artery, damaging the muscle and leading eventually to a myocardial infarction (commonly called a *heart attack* in lay parlance). In its early stages, the occurrence of such an event is called *acute coronary syndrome* (ACS). During ACS, treatment is aggressive to prevent progression to myocardial infarction, as described below.

SYMPTOMS OF CAD

The presence of plaque alone does not cause symptoms of heart disease, such as chest pain, nor does it cause heart damage. Most of the time, even significant blockages do not cause immediate problems. About 75–80 percent of an artery has to be blocked before flow of blood through it is significantly reduced. The majority of people, even those with severe CAD, have absolutely no symptoms and the disease remains silent for many years. The underlying disease may declare itself quite suddenly when the person drops dead with no prior symptoms. Actually, *sudden cardiac death* (SCD) is often the first "symptom" of CAD. Sudden cardiac death is defined as death occurring with cardiac symptoms lasting less than one hour. This time period is, in some cases, extended to 24 hours when death has been unexpected and is unobserved and the diagnosis cannot be made with precision.

The usual cause of SCD is a rhythm called *ventricular fibrillation* (VF) that causes cardiac arrest. This condition is fatal if not electrically reversed by a defibrillator. In the patient discussed in this chapter's case study, we knew he had CAD and he was successfully operated on after the onset of symptoms with relief. However, he may have had blockages that progressed after surgery, or his grafts may have become blocked. Alternately, he may not have had ischemia or myocardial infarction, but rather could have developed ventricular fibrillation that was fatal. Like many patients with CAD, the underlying heart muscle may have been electrically unstable and could have progressed directly into ventricular fibrillation. His death is what is known as an *anniversary death,* as it coincided with two important anniversaries that were related to his wife. Anniversaries of important life events have been shown to be important emotional risk factors in myocardial infarction and sudden death. Such anniversaries include birthdays, marriages, deaths of close relatives, and other significant ceremonial events.

If the artery is severely blocked, the heart does not pump efficiently because it lacks oxygen. This condition is called *ischemia,* meaning a lack of blood flow to heart muscle. The person may experience symptoms due to lack of oxygen and nutrients to the heart and the rest of the body. These symptoms include fatigue, sleepiness, shortness of breath, and/or discomfort in the chest (*angina*), during walking, exercise, or emotional stress. These symptoms occur because there is not enough blood, and therefore oxygen, getting to the rest of the body to support ordinary activities. During such episodes, heart rate and blood pressure increase and there may be perspiration. When the person rests, or sits up from the lying position, oxygen demand decreases, and the heart rate and blood pressure decline to more normal levels after several minutes.

Angina is reversible and can recur whenever the demands for oxygen increase during physical or emotional stress. Angina is felt as a slight or severe discomfort in the chest, throat, shoulders, or arms. Because it may radiate to the pit of the stomach and be felt under the lower sternum, angina can be mistaken for indigestion. Sometimes it radiates to the back between the shoulder blades, or to the lower jaw, where it can be mistaken for a toothache. Many a tooth has been pulled for this reason. If the pain occurs above the lower jaw or below the belly button, it is extremely unlikely to be angina. If a person has discomfort or pain between the lower jaw and the umbilicus, the diagnosis of angina should always be considered as a possibility. Death from angina alone is uncommon, and the person may have many bouts of angina with no damage to the heart. However, ischemia can cause electrical instability and lead directly to ventricular fibrillation and sudden death, as described above.

During stable angina there is usually no damage to heart muscle, and it is similar to a muscle or stomach cramp. In some cases, angina may go on for an hour or more, and occur at rest, even with no exertion. This is called *unstable angina* and requires urgent attention. In such cases, there is slight damage that could progress to a full-blown myocardial infarction with more extensive damage. The person needs hospitalization with an evaluation that includes an EKG, blood tests, and often a cardiac catheterization. Blockages need to be treated with medications, angioplasty or cardiac surgery.

In other cases, a myocardial infarction may come on suddenly with no preliminary anginal symptoms. The person experiences crushing central chest pain, sweats, and may become severely short of breath. These symptoms are classic for what is often called a "heart attack." A heart attack is a lay term that means that there has been real damage to the heart, and it is technically called a *myocardial infarction*. This condition requires immediate hospitalization, bed rest, cardiac testing, and treatment, as described above for *unstable angina*. The difference between unstable angina and the beginnings of a myocardial infarction comes down to a matter of degree on a continuous spectrum of the amount of damage to the heart muscle.

During unstable angina (also known as acute coronary syndrome or ACS) and myocardial infarction, there are characteristic EKG changes that are diagnostic. In ACS, the EKG shows new T-wave inversion followed by new ST-segment depression. These changes indicate that there has been recent occlusion of a coronary artery, reducing blood flow to the heart muscle. The particular cluster of EKG leads that show changes indicate the region in the heart the damage is occurring. If treatment aborts progression, the condition is called a *non-ST elevation myocardial infarction* (NSTEMI).

If the condition progresses, there is ST-segment elevation indicating more damage to heart muscle, and new Q-waves emerge after several hours. The emergence of Q-waves on the EKG indicates that full-thickness damage to the myocardium has occurred, extending from the epicardium to the endocardium.

This kind of damage is called an *ST-elevation myocardial infarction* (STEMI). The location of the Q-waves on the EKG indicates the location of the myocardial infarction (e.g., an anterior wall infarction, or an inferior wall infarction).

When heart muscle is damaged, there is electrical instability of the heart's tissue as a result of disruption of the normal electrical process that keeps the heart beating normally. Such *electrical instability* may continue undetected with the heart beating normally for a long time. But one day, ventricular fibrillation results from increased oxygen demands from very heavy exercise or from emotional stresses caused by the action of adrenaline on the heart. Slight increases in electrical instability can lead to abrupt disruptions in the normal electrical functioning of the heart and subsequently to chaotic and uncoordinated depolarization of the heart. In such cases, the person dies suddenly from ventricular fibrillation, as described in the case study patient. Even when heart muscle damage is extensive, death does not occur unless there is ventricular fibrillation leading to cardiac arrest.

Another form of death occurs during myocardial infarction when the heart muscle is badly damaged by a large infarction. Because of extensive damage, there is global ischemia and the heart gradually slows down and stops beating completely (*asystole*), resulting in death. Very rarely, the heart may actually rupture if there is extensive damage to the ventricular muscle. Death follows rapidly due to blood shooting out of the heart and into the pericardium or chest cavity. If the rupture is small and blood is contained within the pericardial cavity, it is theoretically possible to open the chest and repair the tear. However, in most cases, there is insufficient time to attempt such repair, and many patients will die before this can be done.

DIAGNOSIS OF CAD

The diagnosis of CAD is made every day in doctors' offices, emergency rooms, and hospitals. The suspicion of CAD is raised when someone says he has symptoms of chest tightness, chest discomfort, or pain on exertion, or if there are symptoms of "indigestion." CAD may be chronic or manifest itself suddenly with acute chest pain. In chronic CAD, the patient is asymptomatic or has only mild angina, and there is an opportunity to evaluate the person as an outpatient so that diagnostic testing can be done on an ambulatory basis. When the patient develops the acute onset of chest pain, hospitalization is necessary for both diagnosis and treatment. In the latter case, the patient has either unstable angina or is in the early stages of a myocardial infarction.

The first step in diagnosis is to take a medical history and perform a physical examination. The history is more important than the physical examination as the latter is most often normal in most cases. However, the medical history in classical angina, if well taken, can often make a diagnosis even before cardiac testing is done. If the initial clinical evaluation suggests CAD, the doctor will proceed to perform certain cardiac tests. The details of the most common tests are discussed in detail in Chapter 8.

The difference between testing for stable CAD and more acute conditions such as unstable angina and myocardial infarction is that in the latter cases, the testing takes place in the emergency department and as an inpatient so that rapid treatment can be given to abort progression of a heart attack. The correct order of tests depends on the clinical presentation and what the initial EKG and blood tests show. If this screening shows that the person is not in the throes of an acute coronary syndrome or myocardial infarction, testing can be done as an outpatient with an exercise stress test and echocardiography. If the EKG and cardiac enzymes show the early stages of an active destructive process, the patient is hospitalized and cardiac testing takes another pathway that will not include a stress test, but may include cardiac catheterization.

Here is a guide to how a doctor may proceed in order to make a diagnosis of CAD:

- A baseline EKG is performed to record changes that may help to determine if the chest pain is originating from the heart. This may provide an immediate diagnosis if the person is having serious symptoms of unstable angina or myocardial infarction. In stable angina, there are often no EKG changes in between episodes of chest pain.
- Blood is drawn to check if the person is in the middle of an episode of unstable angina or a myocardial infarction. Myocardial cells contain enzymes (creatine kinase, lactic dehydrogenase, troponin, and myoglobin) that are released when they are damaged. These enzymes will indicate if there is heart muscle damage during unstable angina, ACS, or myocardial infarction. If the EKG and blood tests are normal, the person proceeds to the next stage of testing. If they are abnormal, the patient is admitted to hospital for treatment.
- In otherwise stable patients, an exercise EKG, also known as an exercise stress test, will show how the heart responds to graded increases in exercise when oxygen demand escalates gradually. In the presence of CAD, the stress test often shows changes of ischemia on the EKG.
- An exercise stress test with cardiac imaging (thallium stress test) is done. This test involves a radioactive substance that is injected into the bloodstream to show how much blood reaches heart muscle. It does not actually

show the blockages in the coronary arteries. X-ray images can show if areas of the heart muscle are damaged or "dead." Another related test is Positron Emission Tomography (PET scan) that shows which areas of the heart muscle are healthy and which areas are not.

- Another form of cardiac imaging done during a stress test is echocardiography, which uses sound waves to produce an image of the heart to see how the heart muscle and valves work during exercise stress. The coronary arteries are not seen in this study. If there is ischemia, the heart muscle will be seen to buckle during exercise stress. There may occasionally also be valvular malfunction during exercise stress.

- If the patient has active ischemia and has EKG and cardiac enzyme changes, the diagnosis is *acute coronary syndrome* (ACS) and the patient is hospitalized for further management.

- If ACS is diagnosed, the patient is treated with medications and cardiac catheterization and coronary angiography are performed in the cardiac catheterization laboratory. Radiographic dye is injected into the coronary arteries and high-speed filming of the beating heart is done with X-rays. This resulting movie is called a *coronary angiogram* that shows the actual location, extent, and number of blockages in the coronary arteries. This is the definitive test to make a diagnosis of CAD, and it helps guide treatment, with medications, angioplasty, or surgery.

TREATMENT FOR CAD

CAD is eminently treatable with a variety of methods. Once the diagnosis is made by stress testing or by cardiac catheterization, appropriate treatment should be given. Such treatment for CAD includes an appropriate diet, exercise, medications, angioplasty with or without stenting, and bypass surgery. There are basically four groups of treatments that are prescribed in treating CAD:

1. Lifestyle changes
2. Medications
3. Percutaneous coronary interventions
4. Surgical treatment

These treatments are described below, and it is noteworthy that they are not mutually exclusive. Lifestyle changes, which include diet and exercise, are recommended with both medical as well as with surgical treatment. Even with surgical treatment, medications may also be prescribed depending on the nature of the patient's medical condition. In all cases, however, diet and exercise are fundamental to maintaining optimal health even after direct intervention to correct coronary obstructive disease has been accomplished.

Medical Treatment

Medical treatment, as opposed to surgical treatment, refers to the use of medications, diet, exercise, and stress reduction in controlling the symptoms of CAD and in the prevention of sudden cardiac death from heart disease. Angina due to CAD is classified as *stable angina* when the person is not at immediate risk for a myocardial infarction, and *unstable angina* when the process may progress to a myocardial infarction with damage to heart muscle. Unstable angina is associated with progression of chest pain, often resulting in EKG changes and cardiac enzyme leaks due to heart muscle damage. This condition is called *acute coronary syndrome* and is a medical emergency that requires immediate and aggressive treatment to prevent progression to a full-blown myocardial infarction. It is important to recognize that this process is actually a continuum, so that early treatment prevents progressing to a full-blown myocardial infarction. Though the myocardial infarction itself may be aborted before it actually occurs, some EKG and cardiac enzyme changes do occur.

Treatment of Stable Angina

In most cases of mild *stable angina*, treatment with aspirin is started for prevention of future heart attacks. Aspirin decreases stickiness of platelets. Platelets have a role in clot formation as described earlier, and this contributes to the occurrence of heart attacks. Aspirin treatment prevents clumping of platelets to inhibit clot formation inside the coronary arteries. Though there is a small risk of bleeding with aspirin, especially in the brain, this risk is less than the benefit derived from preventing a myocardial infarction and sudden death.

Nitroglycerine tablets under the tongue provide almost immediate pain relief. The person suffering from CAD should always carry this medication, as angina is unpredictable and may come on at any time, especially with effort or during emotional stress. Nitroglycerin can also be used as a spray, an ointment, or as a sticky patch applied to the skin. Longer-acting nitrates (e.g., isosorbide dinitrate) are also available for continuous and ongoing control of angina.

For more reliable and continuous treatment, drugs called *beta-adrenergic blockers* (also called beta blockers), such as metoprolol, propranolol, and nadolol, are used. These drugs block the action of adrenaline on the heart. By reducing blood pressure and heart rate and the contractile function of heart muscle, physical stress on the heart and oxygen consumption by heart muscle are reduced. These actions of the drug on the cardiovascular system prevent angina and myocardial infarction. These drugs also quite dramatically reduce the rate of sudden death from cardiac arrest.

Other drugs such as *calcium channel blocking agents* (e.g., nifedipine and diltiazem) also help to reduce angina. These drugs relax the smooth muscle in the walls of the arteries, allowing greater blood flow through the coronary arteries. However, this class of drugs does not reduce the rate of sudden death in people with heart disease. The role of so-called "polypills," which are a combination of aspirin, a beta-blocking agent, and a cholesterol-lowering drug such as a statin, is controversial. It is unclear if using such pills, though convenient, is a proper approach to treating CAD, and they are probably best avoided.

Medical treatment for stable angina along with risk factor modification has been shown to be extremely beneficial in controlling symptoms and extending life. There is little evidence that invasive treatment with angioplasty and stenting or surgical treatment with coronary bypass surgery is superior to medical treatment for chronic stable angina pectoris even in the presence of significant blockages in the coronary arteries. This surprising finding may be due to the fact that as the coronary arteries become gradually blocked over many years, collateral channels open up around the blocked arteries. These ancillary blood vessels provide an extensive network of small arteries that feed the heart muscle with blood. This situation is very different from blockages that occur more acutely.

However, in certain cases, such as left main coronary artery stenosis, proximal left anterior descending coronary artery stenosis, and severe three-vessel CAD, angioplasty and/or bypass surgery is the treatment of choice. In some patients with significant left ventricular dysfunction, bypass surgery may also be more beneficial. However, in all of these cases, the risk/benefit ratio must be considered as other concomitant conditions, such as diabetes, kidney disease, or cerebrovascular disease, will increase the risk for complications and death during invasive treatment and cardiac surgery.

Treatment of Unstable Angina and Myocardial Infarction

Unstable angina occurs when the person develops chest, arm, jaw, neck, or back pain due to CAD that lasts for more than 15–20 minutes at rest. Generally, these symptoms are the result of progressive ischemia that may lead to myocardial infarction and possible sudden death. When angina occurs at rest, it is a serious event that is often accompanied by EKG changes that indicate that active ischemia is occurring and prompt medical attention and treatment are neces-sary. When symptoms of unstable angina progress rapidly, *acute coronary syndrome* (ACS) occurs. This syndrome consists of patients who generally present with chest pain at rest, EKG changes showing ST-segment depression or elevation in-dicating myocardial ischemia or infarction, and cardiac enzyme elevation. Coro-nary angiography in such cases shows acute coronary artery occlusion, often with fresh clot in the culprit artery.

Treatment for ACS includes early dosing with aspirin, heparin, beta-adrenergic blocking agents, and intravenous nitroglycerine. If the patient is at home and develops symptoms, he should take an aspirin and nitroglycerine immediately as these treatments may help alleviate symptoms and prevent rapid progression to myocardial infarction. Aspirin prevents platelet aggregation and clot formation in coronary arteries, and nitroglycerine increases myocardial blood flow through the arteries. If chest pain continues and is severe, morphine is given by injection as it is an excellent analgesic and also provides sedation.

A beta-adrenergic blocking drug given intravenously or orally helps stress and strain on the heart by lowering heart rate and blood pressure, leading to a reduc-tion in the demand for oxygen by heart muscle, and so limits further damage. Such agents may cause severe lowering of heart rate (bradycardia) and result in congestive heart failure if incorrectly dosed. They may also cause bronchospasm and are contraindicated in people with asthma.

The anticoagulant heparin is given intravenously or subcutaneously as this drug blocks clotting within the coronary arteries, and thus prevents progression of the thrombotic process that is assumed to be going on in the culprit artery. Heparin can cause bleeding so that clotting tests need to be done to prevent excessive anticoagulation.

In addition, newer drugs called *glycoprotein agents* are helpful in prevent progres-sion of ACS to myocardial infarction. These agents (abciximab, eptifibatide, and tirofiban) attach to IIb/IIIa receptors on platelets and prevent them from clumping together and thus reduce clot formation in coronary arteries. There is, however, an increased risk for bleeding complications as there is interference with blood clotting mechanisms. In many cases, such treatment "cools down" a very hot process that often progresses to serious heart muscle damage. Aggressive early treatment averts more serious damage to the heart and preserves left ventricular pumping action. Invasive treatment with angioplasty and stenting is necessary if unstable angina progresses and blood tests indicate that significant cardiac damage has occurred.

This type of aggressive management with glycoprotein IIb/IIIa inhibiting agents and invasive treatment with angioplasty and stenting has become the standard for "usual treatment" in the United States. Some critics have com-mented that there is not very strong evidence that all cases of ACS need such early aggressive invasive management as it leads to more complications and is more costly than medical management alone. However, in a very demanding and litigious culture as in the United States, it is often hazardous not to be aggressive in treating medical emergencies. In many other countries, unless there is progression of symptoms, the standard approach is conservative management with bed rest, medications, watchful waiting, and vigilance.

Restoration of coronary blood flow in myocardial infarction patients can be accomplished pharmacologically with *fibrinolytic therapy* using agents such as streptokinase or tissue plasminogen activator (TPA). These agents break down fresh clot within the coronary arteries, a process known as *fibrinolysis*. The most critical variable in achieving successful fibrinolysis is time from symptom onset to drug administration. Fibrinolytic therapy is most effective within the first hour of symptom onset, and it can be used for patients who are seen in hospital with a STEMI within the first 12 hours.

Contraindications to fibrinolytic therapy include a history of known blood or coagulation disorders, presence of brain hemorrhage, ischemic stroke, closed head injury within the past three months, presence of some cancerous tumors, signs of an aortic dissection, or active bleeding from ulcers. Fibrinolytic therapy is not commonly used in the United States, where there is a strong preference for invasive treatment with coronary angioplasty and stenting. Fibrinolytic therapy is more commonly used in many European countries and the rest of the world, as it is more cost-effective than invasive treatment. However, it is a useful treatment in communities that do not have easy access to an interventional cardiologist. As a class, the plasminogen activators have been shown to restore normal coronary blood flow in 50–60 percent of STEMI patients. The successful use of fibrinolytic agents provides a definite immediate and long-term survival benefit over years.

An angiotensin converting enzyme (ACE) inhibitor or, less commonly, an angiotensin receptor blocker (ARB), is also started orally in patients with an STEMI. Such drugs, as described in more detail in Chapter 5, block critical biochemical pathways and reduce blood pressure. This effect is useful in reducing strain on the left ventricle, helping it to heal more quickly. After a myocardial infarction, the left ventricle undergoes a process known as *remodeling,* which results in changes in size shape and function. The affected area becomes thin and balloons outward, and healing turns damaged muscle into scar tissue. The ACE inhibitors reduce remodeling so that the healing ventricle tends to retain a more normal shape and size that resemble its original form. The scar is smaller and more compact, thus helping to preserve left ventricular function.

The role of starting a statin drug to lower cholesterol in patients with ACS, regardless of whether the patient has a high cholesterol level, has been debated.

Based on a study called PROVE IT-TIMI-22, it was recommended that patients with ACS be started immediately on 80 milligrams of atorvastatin (Lipitor) daily. The results of this study suggested that deaths, myocardial infarction, and revascularization procedures were reduced by at least 14 percent in the atorvastatin treated group. While the results of this study are impressive, critics have challenged this type of treatment as being unduly aggressive as the long-term safety of such a high dose of drug is unknown. There is a significant risk of muscle or liver damage with high doses of statin drugs. In addition, in early 2012, the Food and Drug Administration sent out an advisory that statins might increase the occurrence of Type 2 diabetes, memory loss, and confusion. Given that it takes years in the case of many drugs to establish both safety and a definitive benefit, it is probably wiser to await further studies before dosing all patients who suffer ACS or myocardial infarction with high doses of statins regardless of whether the low density lipoprotein (LDL) cholesterol level is elevated or not.

The primary objective of medical treatment is to limit muscle damage during the early phases of ACS. The reason this is important is that long-term survival after a myocardial infarction is directly linked to the state of the left ventricle after the person recovers from the myocardial infarction. If the ejection fraction is preserved and is higher than 40 percent, the person does well and can survive with a much longer lifespan. In cases where the left ventricular ejection fraction is reduced to below 40 percent, not only is lifespan shortened, but congestive heart failure may result, as discussed in chapter 5.

Percutaneous Coronary Intervention

Percutaneous coronary interventions (PCI) are treatments that require penetration of the skin with a needle (a *percutaneous* approach) to introduce flexible catheters that have a variety of devices attached to their ends into a coronary artery. These devices are used to open blockages in the artery and increase the lumen diameter so as to allow increased blood flow. Though PCI is an invasive method of treatment, it is considered a *nonsurgical* form of treatment. The most common type of PCI is called *angioplasty*, with or without coronary *stenting*. During ACS, if symptoms persist or if there is evidence for heart muscle damage by EKGs and cardiac blood enzyme measurement, cardiac catheterization is performed to determine the location and the extent of blockages in the coronary arteries. In such cases, not only are blockages detected, but in many cases, there is fresh clot overlying atherosclerotic plaque that is responsible for ACS. Invasive treatment is necessary in such cases to dilate the coronary artery and remove clots.

Angioplasty and Stenting

Medications reduce symptoms of angina and improve exercise capacity, but they do not remove the actual blockages in a diseased coronary artery. When angina cannot be controlled with drugs, and in cases where angina is progressing to a myocardial infarction (i.e., *unstable angina*), cardiac catheterization is done to identify the extent of CAD. The procedure known as cardiac catheterization is described in detail in Chapter 8.

If severe blockages are seen on the angiogram, a balloon catheter can be threaded via an artery in the arm or groin and inserted into a coronary artery. There is an inflatable balloon attached near the end of the catheter. When the catheter is placed right up against the obstruction in the coronary artery, inflation of the balloon with radiographic dye crushes the plaque, creating a larger opening through which blood can flow. Radiographic dye is used as the fluid is radio-opaque and therefore its location within the coronary artery can be seen on the X-ray monitor while the procedure is being performed. This procedure is also called *angioplasty*, or by the more specific term *percutaneous transluminal coronary angioplasty* (PTCA). Fresh clot may also be seen in the radiographic images, and this may be suctioned out or crushed by the angioplasty balloon.

When the artery is opened during angioplasty, it may close up again (*restenosis*) soon after PTCA or in the following months with a rate of closure as high as 40–60 percent in the first year following the procedure, especially in those who have recurrence of angina. To delay restenosis, devices called stents are placed as a scaffolding inside the artery following angioplasty to prevent restenosis. The rate of restenosis is reduced to about 20 percent in the first year after stenting, though in most cases the artery may remain open for years. In the United States, about 80–90 percent of patients have stents placed in the artery during PCI; while in Western Europe, the rate of stenting is increasing and approaching that of the United States.

Stents were introduced in the 1980s and are generally made of metal mesh. They are thus called bare metal stents (BMS). Because a BMS is a foreign body, it can cause a fibrous reaction (much like scar formation) that blocks the stent. Since about 20 percent of BMS close off in the first year, new stents were devised with a drug embedded in the wire mesh to delay restenosis. Such stents are called *medicated, coated,* or *drug-eluting stents* (DES). The medications used are sirolumus (rapamycin) or paclitaxel, and stents coated with these agents reduce restenosis to the single digits. These stents release a drug that slows the formation of tissue that covers the stent with endothelial cells (*endothelialization*), thus preventing progressive closure of the stent. However, the delay in this normal process of endothelializaton of the stent can lead to blood clot formation inside the stent, resulting in total blockage and renewed symptoms of chest pain and possible myocardial damage. The process of stent thrombosis occurs early, often in the days and weeks following placement of the device. To prevent this complication, patients are treated with a combination of aspirin and clopidogrel (Plavix) or ticlopidine (Ticlid).

Multiple stents may be placed in different locations in the coronary tree in one sitting. Such treatment relieves symptoms of angina but has not been shown to prolong life, though the quality of life is often improved. It is an open question whether angioplasty and stenting in stable CAD is superior to treatment with medications alone. Given the fact that PCI is not a benign procedure and may lead to serious complications, it is wise to consider the pros and cons of an expensive and invasive procedure that may indeed make matters worse rather than better. There is, however, little debate that in the treatment of acute coronary syndromes, where patients develop progressive symptoms of chest pain with myocardial damage, PCI is the appropriate treatment.

Following PCI, patients can go home the day after the procedure unless complications occur. Complications include dissection or tearing of the wall of the coronary artery, the occurrence of myocardial infarction, cardiac arrest, or, rarely, death. A not uncommon complication is the occurrence of bleeding at the site of percutaneous entry of the needle. Occasionally, major bleeding around the abdominal cavity may occur, and surgical repair of the bleeding artery and evacuation of clotted blood may need to be done.

Atherectomy and Laser Devices

Another procedure, called *atherectomy*, is applied when balloon angioplasty is not possible if there is hard plaque. A high-speed rotating diamond drill or burr on the tip of a catheter is used to shave plaque from the arterial wall like a "roto-rooter" used for blocked drainpipes. The debris from the plaque is washed away or vacuumed into a chamber in the device and removed. Stenting is often performed after atherectomy to keep the artery open.

Lasers can also be used through a catheter that has a metal or fiber-optic probe on the tip to remove plaque. The laser burns away plaque and opens the vessel. Other uses of lasers include *percutaneous transmyocardial revascularization* (PTMR) and *transmyocardial laser revascularization* (TMLR). In the former treatment, a laser beam is delivered through the catheter and used to create tiny boreholes in the heart muscle of the left ventricle. These holes become channels for blood to flow to oxygen-starved areas of the heart. It is thought that the procedure may cause new vessels to form, reducing symptoms of angina.

The second procedure, TMLR, uses lasers to create tiny channels in the left ventricle. Access is through an incision in the left side of the chest. While the heart is still beating, the surgeon uses the laser to make between 20 and 40 tiny one-millimeter-wide channels in the left ventricle. These channels give a new route for blood to flow into the heart muscle, which may reduce the pain of angina. As the procedure is done on a beating heart, a heart-lung machine is not needed.

Though the Food and Drug Administration has approved laser procedures, lasers are only being used on patients who have not responded to other treatments such as medications, angioplasty, or coronary artery bypass surgery. Results are variable, and fewer and fewer laser procedures are being done as the treatment has not been shown to be superior to more conventional procedures.

Coronary Artery Bypass Grafting Surgery

If there are multiple blockages, surgery is often recommended to provide surgical revascularization by bypassing the blockages using vein grafts. This is often a more complete treatment for angina than angioplasty. However, the risks are also higher than medical management or PCI as it involves anesthesia and surgically opening the chest and stopping the heart in order to do a coronary bypass operation.

During coronary bypass surgery, the surgeon removes a vein from the patient's own leg. The vein that is most often used is the saphenous vein (i.e., a very long vein running up the leg from ankle to groin). Vein grafts are used to reroute blood from the aorta to the coronary artery to bypass the blockage. One end of the vein graft is stitched to the aorta and the other end to the diseased coronary artery beyond the site of the blockage. In this way, arterial blood bypasses the blockage and supplies oxygenated blood and nutrients to deprived heart muscle. Vein grafts can remain open for many years and often provide excellent relief from angina when successful. The operation, when successful, is often superior to PTCA for patients with multiple blockages as it provides more complete revascularization and better relief than PTCA and for many more years.

Sometimes the surgeon uses an artery from the upper part of the chest wall (called the *internal mammary artery*) to reroute blood flow in the chest. The artery is dissected free from inside the chest wall and implanted into the coronary artery to bypass a blockage.

Most cardiac surgery is done by placing the patient on a heart-lung bypass machine to keep blood flowing when the heart is put into cardiac arrest to keep it from beating. Today, it is possible to do surgery on the beating heart with special instruments that immobilize the operative field while the graft is being placed.

There are also less invasive bypass surgery techniques. Surgery can be done by an incision between the ribs to access coronary arteries on the front of the heart. This procedure is called *minimally invasive direct coronary artery bypass* (MID-CAB), and it allegedly reduces the risk of complications. The procedure may reduce patient recovery time, which may decrease the cost of surgery. However, the cost of the additional special instruments required for MIDCAB often offsets the cost of decreased length of hospital stay for the patient. Surgical treatment for heart disease is covered in greater detail in Chapter 10.

Lifestyle Changes

In anyone with CAD, it is very important to encourage the person to embark on a healthy lifestyle. This approach includes a diet low in fat and cholesterol, regular exercise, keeping to a weight that is appropriate, and avoiding tobacco use. Since passive smoking is also risky, one should stay away from smokers to avoid secondhand smoke. Risk factors for developing CAD and its prevention are discussed in Chapter 12. There are a large number of fashionable and faddish diets that have been invented for both weight reduction and prevention of CAD. Dozens of books have been written on the subject, but the best advice is from the American Heart Association (AHA; for AHA recommendations, see http://circ. ahajournals.org/content/114/1/82.full).

The basic principles for a prudent diet can be summarized as follows:

1. A diet from all the food groups that is low in saturated fat and cholesterol, by eating lean meat (poultry without the skin), by not adding saturated fat during cooking, and by avoiding fried foods.
2. Avoid foods that contain trans-fats.
3. Reduce red meat intake to three or four times a week, or keep cholesterol intake to less than 300 milligrams a day.
4. Fish at least twice a week; oily fish such as salmon, cod, herring, and trout contain omega-3 fatty acids can help lower risk for CAD.
5. Fresh fruits and vegetables daily as they are high in vitamins, minerals, and fiber and low in calories.
6. Unrefined whole grain foods containing fiber, which can help reduce cholesterol.

7. Choose and prepare foods so that dietary salt intake is less than 6 grams daily as it helps control blood pressure. Avoid processed foods as they contain high amounts of sodium.
8. Vitamins and essential minerals taken as dietary supplements do not provide any additional protection against heart attacks if dietary intake of these nutrients is adequate.
9. No more than one alcoholic drink a day, assuming there are no contraindications to taking alcohol.

Most important of all, *read the labels* on food products, as they will provide useful information on dietary components in prepared foods. Consultation with a dietitian is helpful to establish the calories a person needs daily and the amount of salt and fat that is ideal for a particular person, especially if there are conditions such as diabetes, kidney disease, obesity, or high blood pressure.

Exercise should be done for 30 minutes a day after discussing an exercise prescription with the cardiologist or internist. If the patient has angina with exercise, this condition should be treated adequately before exercising. Exercising in cold weather should be avoided, and snow shoveling and exertion should not be done if there is a documented history of CAD as this may provoke angina and myocardial infarction. Isometric exercise such as snow shoveling imposes extra physical stress on the heart and also increases oxygen consumption. This condition may cause a myocardial infarction if the demand for oxygen outstrips the supply in people with CAD. Dressing warmly in winter is also essential as cold may increase blood pressure, and this effect increases the work of the heart, leading to angina.

Stress reduction has been advocated as a component of lifestyle changes for patients with CAD. Many cardiac rehabilitation programs provide psychological counseling as well as yoga and meditation exercises to help alleviate stress. No specific or formal guidelines exist for such treatments in CAD, but it should be emphasized that based on subjective reports, such programs do benefit patients who have CAD. Benefits include lowering of blood pressure, a sense of relaxation and calmness, and a perception of feeling more healthy. Different programs utilize their own guidelines, and it is recommended that people who are recovering from myocardial infarction or coronary interventions or bypass surgery follow the guidelines established by the program in which they have enrolled.

Coronary Artery Spasm

Angina can sometimes occur in patients who have normal coronary arteries. The coronary arteries have a smooth muscle component in their walls. This layer of muscle allows the arteries to relax and open wider to provide more blood flow, and they can also constrict down to a smaller size. In some people, this tendency to dilate and constrict is overdeveloped and the arteries go into severe spasm, throttling off blood supply. The result may be rather severe and disabling chest pain from angina. Occasionally, an actual myocardial infarction with damage to heart muscle will result. Serious ventricular arrhythmias, including cardiac arrest from ventricular fibrillation, can also occur. In these cases, an angiogram shows little or no blockage. Calcium channel blockers and nitroglycerine will dilate the coronary arteries and often alleviate spasm. However, this treatment is not a cure as spasm will often recur when treatment is stopped.

Coronary spasm may also occur in otherwise normal people as well as those who use illicit drugs such as cocaine, amphetamines, ecstasy, heroin, LSD, butane and possibly marijuana. Many of these drugs, particularly cocaine, heroin, ecstasy, LSD, and butane, are also thought to induce myocardial damage, and this may result in ventricular fibrillation or asystole. Unfortunately, in some people this action will result in cardiac arrest and sudden death. In younger patients who have no obvious risk factors for heart disease, the diagnosis of toxic induction of spasm and myocardial damage should be suspected.

Occasionally, severe psychological stress, such as during bereavement, can cause both spasm as well as cardiomyopathy, as described in Chapter 5. The coronary artery vessels react to stress by squeezing down and shutting off blood supply to heart muscle due to the higher levels of catecholamines (such as adrenaline) that are released. In those cases where an emotional component to spasm is present or suspected, psychological counseling is advised in addition to medical treatment for chest pain.

Follow-up Treatment

After the primary condition has been treated with medications, or with PCI or bypass surgery, the patient is generally seen in the clinic or doctor's office every four to six months after discharge from the hospital for an assessment of therapy. Obviously, an earlier visit is warranted if there is uncontrolled angina or recurrence of symptoms that occur after initial treatment. At the follow-up visit, symptoms are reviewed to assess the efficacy of treatment, and a physical examination and an EKG are also performed. If there are no new or recurrent symptoms, treatment is continued and no changes are made, unless it is deemed that certain medications are no longer needed. Often, many medications that were started in the hospital will not be necessary as the person recovers. Thus, the patient should ask if each and every medication is really necessary if there are no cardiac or other symptoms at the follow-up visit.

Recommendations are made for changes in the program if necessary for new or recurrent symptoms such as chest pain or shortness of breath or fluid accumulation in the legs. The exercise prescription is modified if the patient can exercise at a more strenuous level or, if effort is not well tolerated, reduced activity will be recommended. It is conventional in the United States to do an exercise stress test without nuclear imaging (if the patient is stable and asymptomatic) to assess for exercise capacity at some stage in the recovery process. Testing is often done on an annual basis for patients with CAD. Stress testing is reassuring to the patients as it confirms they can exercise safely without fear of imminent death. Most fitness clubs also require an exercise stress test or a doctor's statement for enrollment in an exercise program.

If the patient has symptoms of recurrent angina, nuclear imaging is done during the exercise stress test to assess for possible new ischemic changes, and appropriate recommendations made. Often, only medication changes are necessary to control angina. However, if the patient has more serious symptoms, it may be necessary to repeat coronary angiography to assess for stent closure or bypass graft occlusion. In such cases, the patient is readmitted to the hospital and the necessary tests performed and corrective action taken. In asymptomatic patients with well-controlled angina, annual visits are often all that is necessary for follow-up evaluation.

SUMMARY

CAD is very prevalent in the Western Hemisphere and increasingly common in developing nations. When CAD is suspected, testing can be done to uncover the diagnosis and treatment offered; and the majority of cases of mild angina can be treated with medications. However, the trend in the United States has been to veer toward invasive evaluation early in the process. Therefore, patients are being increasingly treated with angioplasty or surgery earlier and earlier in the course of the disease. The choice of treatment is determined by the age of the patient, the severity of the disease, and the choice made by the patient and the doctor.

4

Diseases of the Heart Valves

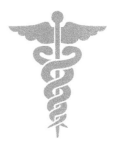

As animals evolved over time, their body size became larger. Such an evolution-ary change required the development of a robust heart that was mechanically efficient and better able to deliver an adequate blood supply with a high oxygen concentration to nourish a larger body size. The fish heart has only two cham-bers: a thin-walled atrium and a thick-walled ventricle that pumps blood around the body. The chambers line up in series and the circulatory system has a rather simple circular path. The atrium squeezes blood into the ventricle that pumps it to the gills, and then on to the rest of the body. Blood returns to the heart after it has circulated through the body of the fish to be pumped around again. The flow of blood is unidirectional and circular as there is no separation within the heart into the venous and arterial systems as seen in reptiles and mammals. Such a linear arrangement of the pumping chambers is the simplest of vertebrate hearts.

The next biological stage in cardiac development is the amphibian heart, with two atria and one common ventricle. Animals such as frogs and toads have three-chambered hearts. Blood from the body returns to the right atrium and passes into the common ventricle. This blood is then pumped into the lungs to pick up oxygen and then returns to the left atrium. The oxygenated blood passes into the common ventricle where there is some mixing with nonoxygenated blood arriving from the right atrium. This lack of separation of the ventricle allows mixing of oxygenated blood with venous blood, thus reducing oxygen saturation from 100 percent to about 70 percent. However, by a process of "streaming," oxygenated blood is pumped into the aorta and to the body, and de-oxygenated blood is pumped into the pulmonary artery. Such streaming provides a functional separation of arterial and venous blood. Such a single-ventricle configuration with an amphibian-like heart occurs in some human congenital anomalies where babies are born with a single ventricle, harking back to an earlier evolutionary period.

In the reptilian heart, there is a partial interventricular septum, so that the common ventricle is divided into a left side and a right side, but they are not quite fully separated. One could call this a "3.5 version" of a four-chamber heart since a connection exists between the right and left ventricular chambers. If a human baby is born with such a heart, it is a congenital defect, as it is really very much like a large ventricular septal defect. However, this arrangement is very convenient in aquatic reptiles as it allows the animal to remain submerged underwater for a long period of time, and for blood to bypass the lungs by shunting it between the ventricles when the animal cannot breathe. A similar situation exists in the human fetus when the lungs are not yet functional, as the fetus is literally swimming in amniotic fluid. Thus, a connection between the atria and/or the ventricles is necessary in fetal life as the heart already begins pumping many months before birth occurs. Closure of the ventricular septal defect occurs after birth so that the heart becomes fully four-chambered in humans and other mammals. In the reptilian heart, in addition to the mitral and tricuspid valves, two additional valves develop at the exits of the two ventricular chambers, as in the mammalian heart.

In mammals, there is a complete separation of the ventricles into the right and left ventricles to produce a true four-chambered heart. This development required the evolution of valves as well for each chamber. As the ventricle pumps there is the possibility that blood coming in from the atria will be pumped back into each atrium. To prevent this, there is a need for a valve between each atrium and each ventricle. As with reptiles, two valves are also present at the exits of the ventricles; thus, the result is a heart with four valves.

The separation into four chambers allows the pressure differentials in each chamber to be preserved in order to keep the heart working efficiently. The evolution of the four valves along with the separation of the heart into four chambers was crucial for maintaining a low-pressure right heart for lung circulation and a high-pressure left heart for systemic circulation to the rest of the body.

THE STRUCTURE AND FUNCTION OF VALVES

A valve is a device that allows for the one-way flow of gases or fluid through a pipe or interconnected tanks or chambers. An ideal valve is one that allows minimal resistance to flow and prevents backward flow or leakage from occurring. Mechanical valves in some machines and pipes are operated externally by hand or electrically. Automatic valves are operated by changes in pressure and flow within the pump or machine itself. In the case of the heart, cardiac valves are operated automatically by the hydraulics of blood flow and by the pressure differentials between chambers. When the chamber pressure is higher, the valves open automatically and when the chamber pressure decreases, the valves close.

The mechanical pumping action of the heart results in pressure differentials between the various chambers so that they open and close depending on whether the heart is in the systolic or diastolic phase of the cardiac cycle. In order to keep blood moving forward, there have to be pressure and volume differentials between the chambers. The valves allow the pressures in each chamber to be maintained within a certain operating range so that the heart can function efficiently.

The mammalian heart has four valves: the *mitral, tricuspid, aortic,* and *pulmonary* valves (see Figure 2.3). The valves between the atria and the ventricles are called *atrioventricular (AV) valves.* The mitral valve has only two leaflets while the aortic, pulmonic, and tricuspid valves have three leaflets (or *cusps*) each. It should be noted that the term "tricuspid" refers to three leaflets. The term applies generally to this feature of a valve but also refers specifically to the tricuspid valve that sits between the right atrium and the right ventricle.

The *mitral valve* lies between the left atrium and left ventricle and the *aortic valve* is located between the left ventricle and the aorta. Similarly the *tricuspid valve* is between the right atrium and the right ventricle, and the *pulmonary (pulmonic) valve* is between the right ventricle and the pulmonary artery. Blood is brought to the heart from the vena cava into the right atrium (RA), and then passes through the tricuspid valve into the right ventricle (RV) to exit through the pulmonary valve. The valves function as the main control points for flow of blood, and they form four major *chokepoints* if they become damaged in any way. Their malfunction can have serious consequences, as will be described later.

String-like tendons attach the edges of the tricuspid and mitral valves to muscular protrusions in the ventricles. These tendons are called *chordae tendinae*. They tether the valve leaflets to the *papillary muscles* (the protrusions in the ventricles). The *chordae tendinae* function as guy lines, which hold a mast, sail, or tent in place, so that the valve leaflets do not get blown backward into the atria when the heart contracts forcefully against the underside of the valve.

The valves themselves are made of thin, flat, semitranslucent flexible membranes called *cusps*. The two cusps of the mitral valve are roughly semicircular. The tricuspid, aortic, and pulmonary valves have three leaflets each and each cusp is roughly triangular. Each leaflet fits snugly with another so that when closed, they form a seal. The valve leaflets are attached to a circular ring called the *annulus*. Various diseases can affect the valve leaflets, the annulus, the chordae tendinae, and the papillary muscles, causing valvular malfunction.

The sequence of events that link the electrical activities of the electrocardiogram (EKG) to the mechanical actions of the heart is best shown in the so-called Wiggers diagram. The pressure-volume curves and the electrical action of the heart were originally overlapped and correlated by Carl J. Wiggers (1883–1963). He was a very well-known American scientist at Western Reserve University (now Case Western Reserve) in Cleveland, Ohio, who obtained his MD at the University of Michigan and studied in Munich, Germany. Wiggers made many important discoveries in cardiac physiology, including the electrophysiology of ventricular fibrillation.

This diagram is a chart that helps cardiologists measure pressure and volume relationships in the heart when the valves open and close as the heart pumps. The chart is created in the catheterization laboratory with catheters placed in the atria, the right and left ventricles, the pulmonary artery and the aorta so that simultaneous pressure tracings can be taken at the same time as the EKG is being measured.

The mechanical action of the heart as it pumps and the intracardiac pressures are usually measured by placing a catheter in only three basic locations: the aorta, the left ventricle, and in the pulmonary wedge position that reflects pressure in the left atrium. Each catheter is connected to a pressure transducer that transforms hydrostatic (fluid) pressure into an electrical impulse that can be recorded on paper as a mechanical waveform traced by a stylus. Because the actions of the heart are known, certain conclusions can be made about what the patterns of these curves represent. At the intersection of the different curves, when intracardiac pressures change, the valves open or close at various points.

When the ventricles start filling with blood from the atria, the mitral valve is open in diastole, and the aortic valve is closed. When the ventricles are full, the amount of blood they hold is called the *end-diastolic volume* (EDV) as already described in Chapter 2. The mitral valve floats upward at the end of diastole and begins to gradually close. When the ventricles start contracting in systole, the mitral valve snaps shut, preventing backward leakage into the left atrium. At the same time, this contraction also forces the aortic valve open, allowing blood to be forcefully ejected into the aorta from the left ventricle.

During contraction, the left ventricle empties blood into the aorta in the time period that represents all of systole. After the blood has left the ventricle, it begins to relax and the aortic valve snaps shut. At this point there is still some blood left in the ventricle, the end-systolic volume (ESV). The difference between the EDV and the ESV is called the *stroke volume* (SV). The stroke volume is the amount of blood ejected with each heartbeat. The mitral valve opens again, allowing blood from the atrium to escape into the ventricle to refill it again. This cycle is then repeated with each heartbeat, allowing an ebb and flow of blood to occur and pushing blood in a forward direction. This phasic flow of blood is what produces the sensation of a pulse felt in the wrist or neck. If any of the valves malfunction severely, the EDV, ESV, and SV of the ventricle are eventually affected. Basically, the same sequence occurs in the right side of the heart, albeit at lower pressure values.

Serious disease of the valves affects many different functions of the heart. Let us take the case of aortic stenosis. The aortic valve becomes narrowed in this condition and forward flow of blood is impeded. To understand how valvular malfunction can affect normal function, Table 4.1 shows the approximate

Table 4.1 Hemodynamic values in a normal heart and in aortic stenosis

FEATURE	Normal	Aortic Stenosis
Heart weight (oz)*	12	16
Number of chambers	4	4
Number of valves	4	4
Number of coronary arteries	2	2
Miles of blood vessels	60,000	60,000
Volume of blood (liters)	5	5
Resting heart rate (beats/min)	70	70
Stroke volume (cc)*	70	55
Ejection fraction (%)*	60	44
Cardiac output (liters/min)*	4.9	4.2
Aortic peak systolic pressure (mmHg)*	120	110
Aortic diastolic pressure (mmHg)	80	80
Left ventricular end-systolic pressure (mmHg)*	120	160
Left ventricular end-diastolic pressure (mmHg)*	5	10
Left ventricular end-diastolic volume (cc)*	120	125
Left ventricular end-systolic volume (cc)*	50	70

Note: An asterisk marks features affected by valve malfunction.
cc = cubic centimeters
mmHg = millimeters of mercury

normal values related to the heart and circulation in the adult, contrasted with the changes seen in aortic stenosis. All of the functional features marked by an asterisk can be affected if the aortic, or other valves, malfunction. In aortic stenosis, the left ventricle enlarges and becomes hypertrophied as it has difficulty pumping blood out into the aorta. The obstruction alters the end-systolic and end-diastolic volumes and pressures in the left ventricle. The systolic pressure differential between the left ventricle (160 mmHg) and the aorta (110 mmHg) is 50 mmHg. This pressure difference is called the aortic gradient. Aortic systolic pressure is also reduced from 120 mmHg to 110 mmHg due to the obstruction to forward flow of blood.

DISORDERS OF THE VALVES

How do valve diseases cause problems? Basically, outside of congenital malformations or malposition, there are two ways a valve can malfunction. It can become narrowed (*stenosis*), or it can leak (*insufficiency*). Narrowing of the valve makes it difficult for blood to flow forward. Improper closure causes leakage of blood backward into the chamber from where it just came. In some cases, both conditions can exist simultaneously. Damage to a valve can involve the leaflets or the annulus. Sometimes, the valve itself is not damaged, but the chordae tendinae or the papillary muscles can rupture, allowing the mitral or tricuspid valve to flap like an untethered sail and causing it to leak blood as the valve can no longer close properly and seal off tightly.

A variety of diseases can cause damage to the valve leaflets. Narrowing of the valve orifice impairs forward flow. Such narrowing is called *valvular stenosis*. If there is leakage due to improper closure of the valve, there is leakage through the opening. Such a condition can occur when the valve is deformed, damaged, or calcified. Improper closure also occurs when the valve ring (annulus) that holds the leaflets in place expands so that the leaflets are too far apart. Disease states such as bacterial endocarditis may erode the cusps, cause perforation, and literally blow a hole in the leaflets, causing leakage as well. This condition of leaking is called *valvular regurgitation* or *valvular incompetence*. Sometimes, both stenosis and regurgitation can coexist in the same valve. In this case, a mitral valve with mitral stenosis may be so deformed by disease that it may leak, causing mitral regurgitation as well.

In valvular stenosis, the valve often becomes thickened and distorted and the leaflets may fuse partially so that they are stuck together. The opening is smaller than normal so that blood does not flow properly from one chamber to the next. This impediment to blood flow causes a high-pressure state to occur inside the chamber that is attempting to empty itself. The accumulation of blood causes the chamber to swell and enlarge progressively over time. Both ventricular size and muscle thickness increase as a result. This condition is called *ventricular hypertrophy*. If impediment to flow is serious, backup of blood leads to accumulation of blood in tissues or in the lungs. Depending on which valves are involved, different symptoms occur and the result is the occurrence of *heart failure*.

CAUSES OF VALVE DISEASE

The aortic and mitral valves are more frequently involved than the tricuspid and pulmonary valves in valvular heart disease. This may be due to the fact that the left heart is a high-pressure system that subjects these valves to greater stresses and strains throughout life, making them more vulnerable to damage.

Both stenosis and regurgitation may occur congenitally or be acquired through various disease states. Valves may naturally become less efficient with age after 70 or 80 years of wear and tear. They may leak or develop calcium deposits, or the chordae tendinae may rupture. Diseases that cause valvular disease include rheumatic fever, infections (endocarditis), various inherited abnormalities of elastic tissue, and toxic substances that weaken heart valve tissue or supporting structures. Some of the major causes of valve diseases are described below.

Aortic Valve Disease

The normal aortic valve has three triangular leaflets that come to a point in the center of the valve so that the commissures when the valve is closed look like a Mercedes-Benz sign. A normal tricuspid aortic valve is shown on the bottom left panel in Figure 4.1. The tricuspid and pulmonic valves also look similar in configuration. Narrowing of the aortic valve occurs due to a congenital bicuspid valve in 40 percent of cases, and in another 50 percent, stenosis is due to aging of the valve. The most common type of congenital valve disease overall is a bicuspid aortic valve. In this condition, the valve has only two leaflets rather than three, as two of them have been joined together. A bicuspid aortic valve is shown in Figure 4.1 in the right lower panel.

Though the bicuspid valve functions normally in early life, it is prone to become thickened and to accumulate calcium later in life. Calcification makes it stiff and narrowed so that a person in the fifth and sixth decades of life can develop valvular stenosis. Aortic valves can become narrowed in later life even if they are not bicuspid. As the valve ages, it deteriorates due to the high pressures it is subjected to as the heart forces blood through it with every heartbeat.

Progressive narrowing of the aortic valve makes it difficult to increase cardiac output during exercise so that there is shortness of breath and even fainting

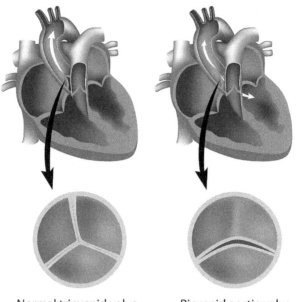

Normal tricuspid valve   Bicuspid aortic valve

Figure 4.1 Heart valves and their locations.
Upper left panel: location of aortic valve. Lower left panel: normal aortic valves showing three leaflets. Lower right panel: bicuspid aortic valve. © Alila07/Dreamstime.com.

when the person exerts himself. If the condition progresses, the ventricle cannot sustain its pumping action and left ventricular systolic and diastolic pressures progressively increase. Eventually, congestive heart failure occurs. In some cases, there is angina during exertion due to the fixed cardiac output and the increased demand for oxygen.

Once congestive heart failure sets in, the mortality rate for severe aortic stenosis is 50 percent in the first two years. If angina occurs, the mortality rate is 50 percent over the next five years. These two symptoms are serious indicators that aortic stenosis needs early surgical correction, and the valve requires replacement with an artificial valve to relieve stenosis. Since the patient is often over the age of 60, the valve of choice is often a porcine valve so that the use of anticoagulation to prevent clots can be avoided.

In Turner syndrome, several congenital abnormalities may coexist. This disorder is genetically inherited in which one of the two sex chromosomes is missing. Typically only one X chromosome is present so the person is XO instead of XX or XY. The person may be born with a bicuspid aortic valve and narrowing of the aorta in the chest, a condition known as *aortic coarctation.*

Aortic insufficiency occurs when there is dilation of the aortic root in hypertension, in Marfan syndrome, in rheumatic heart disease, or when the left ventricle becomes excessively dilated. These conditions result in stretching of the aortic ring, leading to a valve that, when closed, leaves spaces between the leaflets and causing it to leak.

Pulmonary Valve Disease

Pulmonary valve stenosis may also occur congenitally, but this is much more rare than aortic stenosis. The condition is often discovered only later in life if it is an isolated finding and not associated with other types of heart diseases. If the valve is seriously narrowed, right-sided heart failure may occur. Treatment is necessary with valve dilation or replacement if in such cases.

Mitral Valve Prolapse

Mitral valve prolapse is the most common valve disorder in humans, and it is estimated that about 2–3 percent of people have this condition. The actual cause is unknown but it is seen more frequently in connective tissue disorders such as Marfan syndrome and Ehlers-Danlos syndrome.

Prolapse is seen rather frequently on echocardiography where one of the cusps of the mitral valve bulges into the left atrium during ventricular systole. However, some degree of prolapse is often seen even in normal valves and in such cases, this condition is not considered pathological. This condition is also called *floppy valve syndrome* or *Barlow's syndrome*, after John B. Barlow from South Africa, who first described it in 1966.

In mitral prolapse, one or both cusps of the mitral valve are stretched excessively and become floppy and redundant. When the heart contracts, the valve bulges into the left atrium. Because of the deformity of the valve, it will not close snugly, causing backward leakage of blood into the left atrium. If prolapse is excessive, there is frank mitral regurgitation with a large flow back into the atrium, causing enlargement of that chamber. In some cases, the chordae tendinae also become stretched, which makes the prolapse worse. If the chordae burst, as rarely occurs, the leaflet flails into the left atrium and a very loud regurgitant murmur is heard. If the rupture occurs suddenly, the person rapidly develops congestive heart failure due to excessive fluid in the lungs, and death may occur.

Usually there are no symptoms in the majority of patients with mitral valve prolapse. Some patients experience shortness of breath, palpitations, atypical chest pain, and in some cases, atrial arrhythmias. Sudden death is rare, and may be coincidental rather than directly attributable to the prolapsed valve.

In severe cases, surgery is needed to repair the valve by cutting off excessive valve tissue and tightening the chordae to hold the valve in place. This can be done today using a minimally invasive process through a small chest incision, which is sometimes assisted by a robot.

Due to the possibility of infective endocarditis in mitral valve prolapse, antibiotic prophylaxis is recommended before invasive or surgical procedures, as described in the section below on infective endocarditis.

Marfan Syndrome

Though rather rare, this disease is well known to physicians. Jonathan Larson, the 35-year-old Pulitzer Prize–winning author of the rock musical *Rent,* tragically died of undiagnosed Marfan syndrome in 1996, the night before his show opened in New York City. He was seen at two hospital emergency rooms, and his chest pain was misdiagnosed as indigestion and a viral syndrome. He eventually died of a burst aortic aneurysm.

Patients with Marfan syndrome are unusually long-limbed with long tapering fingers. It is an inherited disorder of connective tissue carried by the FBN-1 gene in which a protein called *fibrillin-1* is affected. In this case, because elastic tissue is defective, there is a rupture in the middle layer of the aorta that then starts to balloon out. It results in a tear in the intima, the inner layer of the aorta, which allows blood to get into the wall of the aorta, so that it splits the vessel lengthwise. The expansion is caused by blood getting into the middle layer of blood vessels and results in aortic aneurysm formation.

The expansion of the aorta splits the aorta lengthwise. This condition is called *aortic dissection.* Dissection can start anywhere in the aorta and track forward down into the abdomen. The dissection process can track backward into the root of the aorta and involve the openings of the coronary arteries. If the coronary artery openings are affected, there is blockage of blood flow to the heart, and chest pain develops. This is probably the condition that Larson developed.

Another problem is that the dissection tracking backward also causes expansion of the aortic root, which stretches the aortic ring holding the aortic valve. This stretching results in the valve being unable to open normally, causing leakage to occur. If the diagnosis is accurately made, the aorta needs to be replaced with a graft, and the valve replaced with an artificial valve.

Ebstein's Anomaly

In this congenital condition, the right side of the heart is affected. The tricuspid valve is abnormally shaped and does not move normally. The valve sits deep down in the ventricle as the atrium is very large and the right ventricle very small and weak. As a result of these abnormalities, the valve cannot open and close correctly, and blood leaks backward into the atrium. There is also an atrial septal defect (ASD) and often there are arrhythmias. These conditions overload the right side of the heart. Over time, the enlarged right side of the heart becomes weaker and heart failure develops. Surgery is needed in severe cases, with closure of the ASD and replacement of the valve.

Rheumatic Heart Disease

In the Western world, until the middle part of the 20th century, the commonest cause of valvular heart disease was rheumatic fever. Improvement in living conditions, less crowding, and better nutrition of children have led to virtual elimination of this condition. However, rheumatic heart disease (RHD) is still widespread in developing areas such as in Africa, India, China, Southeast Asia, and South America. Rheumatic fever is caused by streptococcal infections of the throat or following scarlet fever, leading to an abnormal immunological reaction. The bacterium that causes this condition is a special type called Group A beta-hemolytic streptococcus.

The streptococcus does not attack the valves directly in rheumatic fever. Rather, the body forms antibodies in response to the bacteria. These antibodies then attack valve tissues, bone joints, skin, and sometimes brain tissue. Typically, children between the ages of 6 and 15 are the ones most affected, with a lower prevalence among adults. About two to three weeks after the acute bacterial infection, the person develops arthritis of the large joints. There also may be a skin rash and skin nodules. Some patients develop involuntary jerky movements, called *chorea*, due to the antibodies affecting brain tissue.

The heart valves suffer the most damage, and the skin lesions and chorea are really not the problem. Repeated streptococcal infections cause more and more damage to the valves. This process most often affects the mitral and aortic valves. The most common condition is *mitral stenosis* followed by *aortic stenosis*. In more advanced cases, the valves may have both stenosis and regurgitation at the same time.

The damage to the valves affected by RHD results in shortness of breath, progressive cardiac enlargement, and the development of congestive heart failure. Surgery is needed to correct valvular defects that are severe. The valves are also more susceptible to an infection called infective endocarditis.

Infective Endocarditis

Endocarditis is a serious infection of the heart caused by blood-borne bacteria. Though it is often referred to as *subacute bacterial endocarditis* (SBE), it is actually mostly an infection of the valves rather than the endocardium. It occurs when bacteria enter the bloodstream and attach to the surface of the heart valves. This condition is one of the most serious valvular diseases that can occur acutely, as it is life-threatening and can also be very difficult to treat.

In SBE, bacteria attack the heart valves, causing growths on the valve called *vegetations*. These vegetations can be seen as clumps on the valves, the chordae tendinae, or elsewhere in the heart. Though normal valves can be attacked, usually bacteria tend to affect valves that are already abnormal, artificial valves, and hearts of patients who have congenital heart disease. The bacteria can erode into the valve tissue, blowing a hole by causing a perforation in the valve.

Scarring of the valve tissue occurs, causing the valve to leak or become stenotic and incompetent, often at the same time. Occasionally, there may be rupture of the chordae tendinae, causing the mitral valve to flail and get blown into the left atrium during ventricular systole. In this case, there is massive regurgitation of blood into the left atrium, and the mitral valve is virtually useless as it is unable to stop free flow backward into the lungs. The patient may become acutely short of breath and suddenly experience heart failure as fluid leaks out into the lungs.

Bacteria such as streptococcus, staphylococcus, enterococcus, and other less common organisms that live on skin and the gut can enter the bloodstream during surgical and dental procedures. Seeding of the valves with bacteria occurs during tooth cleaning, joint replacement, surgical procedures on the bowels and bladder (including colonoscopy and cystoscopy), severe infections, and intravenous drug use. When bacteria from the mouth and gut gain entry into the bloodstream during these procedures, they multiply in the blood, which provides a rich medium for bacterial growth.

This is one instance when diagnosis and treatment have to be swift, as SBE is a life-threatening condition. Early diagnosis and treatment are essential to prevent extensive damage to the valve or valves affected. The diagnosis is made by drawing repeated blood tests and culturing the blood in the laboratory to identify the bacteria causing the infection. Treatment consists of large doses of intravenous antibiotics that may go on for weeks in some cases to completely eradicate the infection.

To prevent this serious infection, antibiotics are given to patients with known valve disease or artificial valves before surgical procedures. Pretreatment with antibiotics is necessary for such patients for dental procedures such as tooth cleaning, tooth extraction, colonoscopy, and some surgical procedures. The drug of choice is amoxicillin, which is a penicillin derivative. For those who are allergic to penicillin, other antibiotics such as clindamycin, cephalexin, and azithromycin are used for prophylaxis.

Connective Tissue Disease

Connective tissue is tissue that is found outside the cells; it forms a matrix that holds tissue together. It is made up of two proteins: *collagen* and *elastin*. In some types of *autoimmune diseases* that are poorly understood, the body makes antibodies against these tissues. This tissue then becomes inflamed, leading to arthritis, swelling of tissues, and generalized pain. Lupus erythmatosus, rheumatoid arthritis, and polyarteritis nodosa can affect the aortic and mitral valves. These diseases generally cause regurgitation. However, pericarditis and myocarditis can also occur in some cases of connective tissue disorder.

Diet and Medications

The use of fenfluramine and phentermine ("fen-phen") as an appetite suppressant for weight loss caused valve problems and death. Fenfluramine causes damage to valvular tissues, resulting in mitral, tricuspid, and aortic regurgitation and pulmonary hypertension. It was withdrawn in 1997 as a result of the toxic and potentially fatal effects on heart valves and the pulmonary circulation.

In late December 2009, the European Medicines Agency recommended the withdrawal of benfluorex, a diabetes medicine related to fenfluramine, because of the risk of heart valve disease. In France, the medication was marketed as Mediator and was on the market between 1976 and 2009. It allegedly caused up to 2,000 deaths and was thus withdrawn.

Radiation Therapy

High-dose radiation therapy to the chest area for cancer can cause heart valve disease. Radiation damage causes fibrosis in normal tissue. Heart valve disease due to radiation therapy may not cause symptoms for as many as 20 years after the therapy ends.

SYMPTOMS AND DIAGNOSIS

The diagnosis of valve disease is most often made during a routine checkup when the doctor hears a murmur, which is a sound made when blood flows though a valve. Occasionally, a parent or a partner hears a whooshing or squeaking sound in the chest and alerts the person or a doctor. The altered flow makes a noise, due to turbulence caused by stenosis or regurgitation. These noises may be low-, medium-, or high-pitched, depending on the kind of valve disease and the type of valve itself. The sounds are so distinctive in most cases that the cardiologist can often make a diagnosis as to the exact valve involved. In some cases, it is possible to make a judgment as to how severe the problem may be and whether the murmur does not deserve further evaluation.

If the valve impedes blood flow, the person experiences shortness of breath, and chest pain or angina occurs in some cases. Fainting, or syncope, occurs in severe aortic stenosis. Congestive heart failure may occur in severe aortic or mitral valve disease. In young patients, there may be failure to thrive and the child appears sickly and wizened.

By piecing together the history and physical examination, the doctor can make a reasonably accurate estimation of the seriousness of the problem at hand. However, diagnostic testing is necessary to make an accurate diagnosis. The plain chest X-ray is not very useful in making the diagnosis of valvular heart disease. The single best test for valvular disease is the echocardiogram, as it is noninvasive, relatively inexpensive, and can be done in less than one hour. This test, when combined with a Doppler flow study, gives the doctor an accurate diagnosis of the actual valve involved and an estimation of the extent of the problem. Calculations can be made using a formula, in the case of aortic stenosis, to estimate the gradient across the valve by echocardiography.

In most cases, cardiac catheterization is necessary to measure pressures inside the heart to measure the degree of valvular malfunction (see Table 4.1). However, in straightforward cases such as pure aortic stenosis, many surgeons are willing to operate based only on the results of the echocardiogram. By collating the results of echocardiography and cardiac catheterization, a decision is made whether the patient should undergo a procedure to correct the condition.

TREATMENT

In most cases, when stenosis or regurgitation is not causing any symptoms, it is not necessary to repair or replace the valve. A natural valve is almost always superior to the best artificial valve when the patient has no symptoms. However, with abnormal valves, antibiotic prophylaxis is always recommended before any non-cardiac surgical procedures.

In cases where the valve is suspected to be causing problems such as shortness of breath, chest pain, or heart failure, cardiac catheterization is necessary to determine the severity of the problem. A decision is then made whether the valve should be cracked open using balloon angioplasty, if it should be repaired surgically, or if an artificial valve should be placed. These treatments are described in Chapter 8.

A variety of mechanical artificial valves and tissue valves are available for replacement if a valve is severely diseased. Valves are mechanical if they are made entirely of metal, silicone, pyrolytic carbon, fabric, and other material. These valves may cause the formation of clots. Therefore, the patient needs to be on blood-thinning medication, known as anticoagulants, after valve replacement.

Tissue valves are made from porcine (pig) valves that are specially treated and sewn onto a ring. Valves can also be made from pericardial tissue from horses and cows. The animal material is sewn onto a strut or ring that holds the tissue in place so that it fits into the position of a human valve in the heart. These animal valves do not require the use of blood thinners in many cases and this is a huge advantage. However, biological valves can become calcified 10 to 15 years after surgery, so they are generally reserved for patients over 65 years old. Very occasionally, a surgeon may take out the pulmonary valve and put it in place of a stenotic aortic valve. This is an ideal solution as the valve will work extremely well, as it is the patient's own tissue that is being used.

There is, of course, operative risk, including death and the fact that the replaced valve may turn out to make things worse. Also, the new valve may get infected during surgery, and this may require a second operation under less than ideal circumstances. Valve replacement is a rather major operation, and careful thought should be given to valve replacement, as mechanical or tissue valves can have problems themselves that may well be worse than the original valve that was malfunctioning.

SUMMARY

Valves regulate the flow of blood to make the heart beat more efficiently. Diseases of the valves impair the proper functioning of the heart and can lead to heart failure. Valvular heart disease is most commonly seen in the mitral and aortic valves. Medications cannot cure diseases of the valves. In cases of severe valvular disease, surgery is most often the best treatment, involving either repairing or replacing the valve.

5

Disorders of the Heart Muscle and Congestive Heart Failure

The myocardium is the main muscular component of both the right and the left ventricles. It occupies the space between the epicardium and the endocardium, as described in Chapter 2. This type of heart muscle is called *involuntary muscle* as its contraction is automatic and not under conscious control, like *voluntary* or *skeletal muscle* that we use for locomotion. There is a third type of muscle in the body called *smooth muscle*, which is also not under conscious control, found in the walls of blood vessels, stomach, intestines, and bladder.

It is the action of the myocardium that propels blood out of the heart, to the lungs and around the body. Obviously, the myocardium's pumping action is continuous throughout life, and if it stops contracting, the person will die rapidly. Though a pacemaker in the atrium controls the normal heartbeat, the myocardiam itself is capable of spontaneous contraction at a rate of about 20 to 40 beats per minute. Unlike other types of muscle in the body, the myocardium is very dependent on oxygen. It actually consumes a huge proportion of oxygen in the blood, second only to the brain.

Severe weakening or damage of heart muscle due to a variety of causes is called *cardiomyopathy*. The commonest cause of damage to heart muscle is myocardial infarction due to coronary artery disease. When extensive damage due to myocardial infarction occurs, there is serious loss of cardiac pumping action. After the heart heals, there is severe dysfunction and the condition is called *ischemic cardiomyopathy*. However, clinically, it is conventional to use the rubric "cardiomyopathy" when referring to loss of contractile function of the heart when the cause is other than coronary artery disease. People with cardiomyopathy are vulnerable to both atrial arrhythmias such as atrial fibrillation, as well as being at high risk for sudden death from ventricular fibrillation.

Weakening of the myocardium leads to reduced pumping action of the heart, resulting in an accumulation of fluid in the lungs and the rest of the body. Reduction in the pumping action of the heart also leads to low blood flow to the kidneys, preventing excretion of salt and water and thus increasing water retention. This condition is called *congestive heart failure* (CHF), or simply abbreviated to *heart failure*.

The term *heart failure* sounds rather frightening to the layperson, but it does not mean a *complete* and *total* failure of the heart to pump. Clinically, the term *failure* means that the heart has failed to keep up with the normal requirements of the body to deliver oxygen and nutrients to the organs due to decreased forward flow of blood. Heart failure is said to be *acute* in onset when it occurs suddenly and death can occur if it is left untreated. This condition occurs if there is an acute injury to the heart after a myocardial infarction or in acute myocarditis. *Chronic* CHF may occur over weeks or months and is generally a permanent condition as the underlying condition may not be easily reversible, even after congestion is treated. After fluid is cleared from the body, the patient is said to be in *compensated congestive heart failure* and will require ongoing medical treatment.

While treatment strategies are similar, acute onset of CHF requires immediate or emergency attention or the patient will literally drown and possibly die from fluid accumulating rapidly in the lungs. When acute heart failure occurs due to excessive fluid administration (e.g., after surgical procedures when the patient is fed intravenously), there is nothing wrong with the pumping action of the heart. This type of heart failure is transient as it is due to fluid volume overload and not due to underlying heart disease. It is fully reversible and the patient recovers completely after the fluid is removed with diuretic therapy.

The number of patients with CHF is increasing as more and more patients are surviving other cardiac conditions that eventually lead to CHF. About 5 million people in the United States have CHF and another half a million people are newly diagnosed each year. Many patients are readmitted to hospital within 6 months, making this a costly disease to treat. It is estimated that $35 billion is spent annually in taking care of such patients in the United States alone. In the United Kingdom, it is estimated that 2 percent of the National Health Service budget is spent on the treatment of CHF.

When the myocardium is affected by a variety of diseases, this results in two very different clinical conditions—*systolic dysfunction* and *diastolic dysfunction*. Both conditions lead to congestive heart failure under certain conditions. In systolic dysfunction, there is loss of muscle tissue so that the heart does not pump normally. The heart can also become dysfunctional without the apparent loss of heart muscle tissue. This condition happens if there is impairment due to increased "stiffness" of the heart muscle when it loses its supple quality, and it fails to relax normally during diastole so that the ventricles do not fill properly with blood. This condition is called *diastolic dysfunction*.

SYSTOLIC DYSFUNCTION

The contraction phase of the myocardium is called cardiac *systole*. Severe damage to heart muscle produces a condition called *systolic dysfunction*. Impairment occurs during contraction because there is not enough heart muscle to meet the demands of the body, and the heart cannot maintain the normal circulation of blood.

Causes

The commonest cause of systolic dysfunction is myocardial infarction. The heart is a surprisingly tough organ and can actually take quite a hit and lose a considerable amount of muscle before any serious malfunction is noticeable. The normal heart has a baseline ejection fraction of 60–70 percent, that is, 60–70 percent of blood is ejected from the left ventricle per heartbeat. A myocardial infarction has to damage the heart muscle and reduce the ejection fraction from the normal baseline to about 40 percent before there is a noticeable difference in performance. Thus, until there is damage to over a third of heart muscle, there is often no noticeable change in function with normal physical activity. Dysfunction of the heart is noticed only when the person is physically active and the heart is abnormally stressed by exercise or fluid overload, leading to shortness of breath or CHF.

Cardiomyopathy is another cause of systolic dysfunction. Cardiomyopathy is classified as *dilated* or *hypertrophic*, depending on the anatomical configuration of the ventricles. In dilated cardiomyopathy, the heart becomes enlarged and flabby due to extensive destruction of heart muscle. In hypertrophic cardiomyopathy, the heart muscle becomes thickened and heavy and contraction is less efficient as a result. Dilated cardiomyopathy is caused by alcohol, certain types of viruses (e.g., Coxsackie B, mumps, measles, zoster, HIV virus), genetic defects, diabetes, postpartum (after delivery of a baby), drugs and alcohol, obesity, chemotherapy for cancer (e.g., adriamycin), heavy metal poisoning, and thyroid disease. Nutritional problems, such as protein malnutrition or deficiencies in vitamin B1 or vitamin D, can also cause this condition. Rare causes include diseases such as amyloidosis, acromegaly, sarcoidosis, and hemachromatosis. In about a third of cases of acute inflammation of the myocardium (*myocarditis*) that leads to cardiomyopathy, no cause is found, though a viral etiology is probably the culprit.

An unusual cause of cardiomyopathy is severe acute psychological stress, such as the sudden loss of a loved one. This condition has also been called *broken heart syndrome*, or *takotsubo cardiomyopathy*. (*Tako-tsubo* is Japanese for a bulbous vessel or fishing pot used to trap octopus.) Often only the apical part of the left ventricle is involved and balloons out in bulbous form. It is presumed that acute psychological stress, such as the loss of a spouse, leads to high levels of adrenaline, and the condition is called *stress-induced cardiomyopathy*. Excessive adrenaline is theorized to drive the heart constantly beyond its tolerance and this allegedly damages the myocardium. Blood pressure decreases due to left ventricular dysfunction as cardiac output decreases due to lack of proper pumping action. Treatment consists of medication for support of low blood pressure and beta-adrenergic blockers to limit the damaging effects of adrenaline. Most patients with stress-induced cardiomyopathy recover fully as the condition is reversible and death is unusual.

Hypertensive hypertrophic cardiomyopathy occurs in people who have hypertension. The inherited form of hypertrophic cardiomyopathy is discussed more fully in Chapter 13. In the case of high blood pressure, the muscle is initially in good shape and will actually become thicker and more muscular to cope with the high pressure against which it has to pump. This condition is called left ventricular hypertrophy as the left ventricle is the most affected part of the heart. Though the myocardial muscle thickens and the ventricle enlarges, it is less efficient than normal. If hypertension is left untreated, this condition progresses and leads to *hypertensive cardiomyopathy*.

In aortic stenosis, the aortic valve impedes forward blood flow, forcing the left ventricle to pump against an obstruction. The increased force mounted by the left ventricle leads to hypertrophy and enlargement of the heart. A similar process happens to the left ventricle when there are leaky mitral and aortic valves where blood leaks backward through the valves, causing the ventricle to pump harder to cope with an increased volume of blood. In all these cases, there comes a point when the left ventricle cannot cope with the higher load of blood it has to handle, and it basically reaches a point when it fails to function normally. This condition results in blood damming back into the lungs, and raising the pressure in the lung circulation. As described below, the excess of blood in the lung circulation results in fluid leaking into the alveoli, causing CHF.

Symptoms

The commonest symptoms of CHF due to either systolic or diastolic dysfunction are fatigue, shortness of breath, cough, and fluid retention. Fatigue is due to lack of blood flow to the body, resulting in an inability to perform normal physical activity. Shortness of breath, cough, and swelling of extremities are due to fluid retention in the lungs and legs. Some patients may become somnolent and mental cognition can be impaired due to fluid retention.

The lungs are made up of millions of thin-walled air sacs called alveoli that are filled with air. The alveoli are coated with capillaries that feed them with blood so that gas exchange takes place by absorbing oxygen and releasing carbon dioxide. The air-filled alveoli offer little resistance to high pressures within the blood vessels, so that plasma seeps out into the alveoli. This condition happens sometimes when the pressure in the capillaries feeding the alveoli exceeds a certain threshold level. The alveoli become congested, the lungs fill up with fluid from the bottom up, and the person becomes progressively breathless. Fluid in the lungs prevents oxygen from entering the blood and into the thin-walled capillaries that coat the alveoli. This situation leads to a condition called *hypoxia*, which refers to a low oxygen level in the blood.

Fluid also backs up into the liver and the lower limbs, resulting in liver enlargement and swelling of the legs. Leg swelling is called *edema* (spelled *oedema* in British English). Fluid can also build up in the abdomen, causing it to swell up gradually, which is referred to as *ascites*. The person puts on as much as 20 pounds of weight and becomes short of breath on walking even short distances. They often cannot lie flat due to congestion in the lungs, using three or four pillow to prop themselves up to breathe more easily. If lung congestion is severe, the person may suddenly wake up in the middle of the night feeling extremely short of breath—a condition known as *paroxysmal nocturnal dyspnea*. Sitting up reduces return of venous blood to the heart, lowering the volume of blood the heart has to pump. When the latter condition occurs, it indicates that CHF is occurring intermittently and there is an urgent need for treatment.

A condition called *cardiac cachexia* occurs when CHF is left untreated. Cachexia means generalized wasting of the body with loss of lean muscle, fat, and bone tissue. Since this condition appears to be independent of the severity of CHF, ejection fraction, and exercise capacity, it is not due solely to the lowering of cardiac output. Cachexia probably results from poorly understood and complex neuroendocrine and immunological reactions. The body produces higher levels of chemicals that affect metabolism such as epinephrine, norepinephrine, cortisol, renin, aldosterone, and inflammatory cytokines in cardiac cachexia. It is thought these chemical substances produce an imbalance between anabolism and catabolism that leads to loss of body tissue, and the patient just wastes away. The outlook for patients with cardiac cachexia is grim, and appropriate treatment strategies have yet to be devised.

Diagnosis

The initial diagnosis of heart muscle disease and CHF is made primarily by the clinical history and by physical examination of the patient. In cases of acute heart failure, it is obvious that the patient is visibly short of breath and there may be blueness of the lips, sweating, and audible wheezing, heard even without a stethoscope.

Blood pressure is often normal, but it is lowered in severe cases of CHF. If the person has hypertension as the underlying cause for CHF, blood pressure is elevated. There is swelling of the legs (edema), and in advanced cases, there is distention of the abdomen (ascites). The heart sounds are altered or muffled, and a third heart sound, called a gallop, is often heard. One or more murmurs may be heard in cases of valvular disease. The lungs show signs of fluid accumulation with crackles in the lung bases audible with a stethoscope, along with wheezing as well if CHF is more advanced. Liver enlargement and ascites is discovered by examination of the abdomen.

Chest X-rays show congestion of the lungs and the heart is often enlarged. In some cases, fluid seeps out of the lungs and into the chest cavity in large amounts that obliterates part of the lungs. This accumulation is called a *pleural effusion*. Removal of fluid is needed if the effusion is large and if it impairs breathing. A large bore needle is stuck into the chest wall, and the fluid is drained from the chest through the needle. Echocardiography shows increased thickness of the ventricular walls in hypertrophic cardiomyopathy, and increases in ventricular volumes in dilated cardiomyopathy. There is decreased heart muscle function with a lowered ejection fraction in systolic heart failure. If there is valvular heart disease, this will also be discovered on echocardiography. In cases where coronary artery disease is suspected, cardiac catheterization is necessary to identify the extent of the disease.

DIASTOLIC DYSFUNCTION

Diastole is the phase in the cardiac contraction cycle when the heart relaxes between beats and fills with blood, getting ready for the next heartbeat. Diastolic dysfunction is due to the loss of normal pliability and suppleness of the heart muscle. The best analogy for diastolic dysfunction is the hardening and weathering of soft leather after being left out in the cold and rain. When the left ventricle is stiff and not pliable, the atria cannot empty completely into the ventricles. This situation allows blood to dam up and fill the lungs with excess blood. The increased volume and pressure in the lungs from the excess blood causes pulmonary congestion and CHF. Excess blood also backs up from the lungs to the right side of the heart and is then transmitted backward into the veins, feeding blood to the right side of the heart and allowing fluid accumulation in the rest of the body. In diastolic dysfunction, the left ventricle often appears to be normal or thickened, but contracting normally on echocardiography, yet CHF occurs. This condition is thus more difficult to diagnose, and often the condition is not clinically manifested as dramatically as in systolic dysfunction.

Causes

The cause of diastolic dysfunction is often unknown, but it usually occurs with increasing age, in diabetes, and in obesity. In conditions such as high blood pressure, hypertrophic cardiomyopathy, and aortic stenosis, diastolic dysfunction is due to thickening of the ventricles. As the myocardium thickens, it cannot pump efficiently due to the heavy muscle mass. Diastolic dysfunction can also occur briefly during periods of transient myocardial ischemia when blood flow to the heart muscle is momentarily interrupted.

Other rare causes of diastolic dysfunction are infiltrative diseases such as amyloidosis, hemochromatosis, sarcoidosis, and glycogen storage disease. In these conditions, abnormal substances such as amyloid, iron, and glycogen become deposited among the muscle fibers of the heart, making the myocardium stiffer than normal.

Symptoms

Diastolic dysfunction leads to much the same symptoms as systolic dysfunction. Symptoms may be disabling in severe cases, and much the same as with systolic dysfunction, but often not as dramatic in onset or as severe. The most prominent symptom is difficulty in breathing, first with exertion and later even at rest. Patients often have fatigue as a prominent symptom with shortness of breath on walking or climbing stairs. A sensation of chest heaviness is quite common, and edema often occurs in these patients. Florid and severe CHF as seen with systolic dysfunction is not common, as left ventricular function is largely preserved. Since there is no really good treatment that is very effective, patients with diastolic dysfunction often never really get better and dyspnea on exertion and fatigue often persist despite therapy.

Diagnosis

The diagnosis of diastolic heart failure is difficult as there are no uniform criteria that are agreed upon. The main method of making this diagnosis is by clinical history, the presence of another concomitant disease, and by echocardiography. The symptoms of shortness of breath, edema, and lung congestion are nonspecific and common to many other cardiac and lung conditions. The echocardiogram shows overall preserved left ventricular systolic function or left ventricular hypertrophy. The Doppler waveform of the mitral valve during echocardiography is used to evaluate blood flow across the valve. In diastolic dysfunction, there is often a distinctive pattern that is helpful in suggesting the diagnosis. In some cases, a cardiac biopsy may be done to establish the diagnosis of amyloidosis, sarcoidosis, or glycogen storage disease. In other cases, there are no distinctive findings, and the diagnosis is made by an exclusionary process.

TREATMENT OF CONGESTIVE HEART FAILURE

Treatment Strategy

The strategy for treatment for both acute onset of CHF and chronically occurring CHF is two-pronged and consists, first, of removing excess fluid and, second, of boosting the pumping action of the heart to improve cardiac output. Specific medication choices depend on the underlying cause of CHF, the acuteness of the problem, and the condition of the left ventricle.

In patients who fill up rapidly with fluid in the lungs, the condition is called *acute* or *decompensated congestive heart failure*. Patients who develop CHF over a period of time and then need to be maintained on medications to control CHF are said to have *chronic* or *compensated congestive heart failure*. The acute onset of CHF requires urgent treatment. In such cases, the patient is rushed to hospital and given high-dose oxygen, delivered via an oxygen mask. Sometimes an endotracheal tube has to be inserted into the windpipe and oxygen delivered directly to the lungs under pressure through a ventilator to oxygenate the blood. Since room air contains only 21 percent oxygen, delivering 40–100 percent oxygen is necessary for a short period of time to tide the person over the acute phase of CHF. The oxygen tension from the ventilator is reduced over time, and then the tube is removed when the person is judged to be able to breathe again on his own.

Excess fluid is removed from the body using a diuretic given intravenously, and then orally. The specific medications are described in detail below. In some cases of acute onset CHF (e.g., in patients where there is fluid overload with little or no myocardial damage), there is no need to continue diuretics on a long-term basis. These patients include those with normal hearts who receive excessive intrave-nous fluid accidentally while in the hospital, or those who have *high output heart failure*. In the latter case, the heart need not be diseased, but is taxed beyond its normal capacity due to severe anemia, hyperthyroidism, beriberi (Vitamin B1 or thiamine deficiency), ateriovenous fistula, or Paget's disease. In the last two cases, there is an increased runoff of blood in the peripheral vasculature that puts an incredibly high demand on the heart.

After immediate treatment with oxygen and a diuretic, measures are taken to increase cardiac output. This is done by giving drugs that either "offload" the heart, or that directly boost the pumping action of the heart. Offloading means gradually reducing blood pressure to relieve strain on the left ventricle to allow increased amounts of blood to be pumped out. A variety of drugs for offloading the heart are described below. Drugs that can boost the contraction of the heart to improve cardiac output are also described later.

The treatment for more chronic forms of CHF is fairly standard and similar to that for acutely occurring CHF. However, in many cases, such patients do not require hospitalization, and most can be investigated and treated as outpatients. The basic problem is that too much fluid has been accumulating in the body over a period of time, and the patient is in no acute danger though he has difficulty in breathing. The aim of treatment is to remove that fluid, and this is generally done with a diuretic, as for the acute onset of CHF. Home care is available in many communities where a visiting nurse can monitor the patient, as this avoids high hospitalization costs.

Medical Treatment for CHF

Diuretics such as a thaizide, furosemide (Lasix), metolazone (Zaroxolyn), bu-metanide (Bumex), and spironolactone (Aldactone) are most commonly used. Other agents may be used to strengthen the heartbeat. In the past, it was stan-dard to administer the digitalis glycosides, digoxin and digitoxin. These drugs strengthen the heart's contractile ability. Due to the risk of toxicity and pos-sible death from cardiac arrest, especially in older patients and those with kidney disease, digitalis drugs have been used less and less in the United States. However, in many other countries, digitalis drugs continue to be used routinely for the treatment of CHF as a cheaper alternative to other drugs. Dobutamine is sometimes given intravenously to increase the contractile force of the heart. Intravenous treatment with a new group of natriuretic peptides such as nesiritide (Natricor) has not been shown to be of benefit. If nesiritide is to be used, it is done so with caution.

A mainstay of treatment for left ventricular dysfunction is a group of drugs acting on the renin-angiotensin system (RAS). These important drugs have made a big difference to the treatment of CHF by improving cardiac output, prompting healing of the left ventricle, and reducing long-term mortality. Originally intended for treatment of hypertension, these drugs work on various chemical pathways in the RAS to lower blood pressure. There are two related groups of drugs working on different parts of the RAS: the angiotensin converting enzyme inhibitors (ACEI) and the angiotensin-II receptor blockers (ARB). Decreasing blood pressure, even when it is normal, actually helps to boost cardiac output. Examples of ACEI are ramipril (Altace) and captopril (Capoten). The group of ARB agents includes valsartan (Diovan) and losartan (Cozaar).

These drugs, however, can make kidney disease worse in many patients, In patients who cannot take these ACEI or ARB because of kidney dysfunction, a combination of isosorbide dinitrate (Isordil) and hydralazine is used to offload the heart. This combination of nitrates and hydralazine has been shown not only to effectively treat CHF, but also to reduce long-term mortality rates.

Though it is counterintuitive, beta-adrenergic blocking drugs are important in left ventricular systolic dysfunction and are often helpful in managing CHF. These drugs depress heart muscle and therefore make CHF worse when given in excess. However, they also decrease oxygen consumption by lowering heart rate and blood pressure, and thus help to control CHF. Carvedilol (Coreg) and metoprolol (Lopressor) are two commonly used beta-blockers in treating heart failure. These drugs, especially when used with ACEI agents, have also been shown to reduce long-term mortality rates by preventing sudden cardiac death. They are thus an essential part of the treatment of patients with left ventricular dysfunction.

In patients with diastolic heart failure, no treatment has been found to be very satisfactory. A group of drugs called calcium channel blockers (CCB) has been used with partial success. These CCB drugs such as diltiazem (Cardizem) and verapamil (Calan) have been found to improve symptoms. The ACEI candesartan has been shown to reduce readmissions for heart failure, but there is not much evidence that these drugs really help very much.

One of the mainstays of treatment for CHF is salt restriction, to avoid retention of water, as salt and water travel together in the body. Salt is also a factor in causing high blood pressure, so salt restriction is very important in such patients. A teaspoon of salt contains about 6 grams of salt. Since salt is made up of 40 percent sodium and 60 percent chlorine, the amount of sodium in a teaspoon is 2.4 grams (or 2,400 milligrams). This amount of salt is the maximum recommended intake for adults. The minimum amount of salt required is about 1.5 grams (1,500 milligrams) a day to replace what is lost in sweat and urine. However, most Americans take in about 3 to 5 grams of salt daily in the diet. Foods such as cold cuts, most processed meat and vegetables, canned, packaged, and fast foods, cheese, chips, ketchup, and soy sauce are very high in salt. These foods and table salt should be eliminated as completely as possible. Without fixing the daily salt intake, a medication program to control CHF will not be effective, especially in people with severe ventricular dysfunction. The reading of food labels and consultation with a dietitian are essential so that the patient is tutored carefully on avoiding foods that contain high amounts of salt.

In patients with alcoholic cardiomyopathy, it is essential that they abstain completely from alcoholic beverages of all kinds. In people who are susceptible to viral infections, influenza vaccine should be given during flu season, though there is no good evidence presently that such vaccination will prevent viral cardiomyopathy.

Invasive Procedures for CHF

Invasive treatment is used in severe cases of CHF when medicines do not alleviate symptoms. When there is massive damage to the left ventricle, cardiac output decreases significantly and the patient develops severe low blood pressure and CHF. This condition is life-threatening and is called *cardiogenic shock*. In these patients, a *counterpulsation device* is inserted through the groin into the thoracic aorta and connected to an intra-aortic balloon pump (IABP). The device that is inserted is a catheter with a cylindrical balloon around it that can be mechanically inflated and deflated using helium. Inflation of the balloon occurs in diastole by synchronizing it with the EKG. Inflation of the balloon increases blood pressure, forcing more blood into the coronary arteries, thus improving circulation to heart muscle. Deflation of the balloon allows more blood to be ejected into the aorta and boosts cardiac output. This method of treatment, though very uncomfortable for the patient, improves circulation to the heart when it is severely damaged supposedly and helps healing of heart muscle. When the heart muscle recovers after several days, the IABP is weaned off and the balloon is withdrawn.

Heparin is used for anticoagulation to avoid clot formation around the catheter. Complications include clotting around the balloon and possible obstruction of blood flow to the legs with the risk of amputation due to gangrene.

Sometimes, extracorporeal membrane oxygenation (ECMO) is used in conjunction with an IABP when oxygenation is suboptimal due to severe heart failure. This process involves placing a catheter in a vein or artery and passing blood through a membrane oxygenator that delivers oxygen to the blood and then returns the blood to the body via another catheter. This method of oxygenation helps the patient after a large myocardial infarction or cardiac arrest, until a ventricular assist device can be placed. This method can also be used together with *ultrafiltration*, as the techniques are similar.

Ultrafiltration is a method to remove excess fluid from the body, and it is done in patients with kidney dysfunction or in those patients where diuretics do not have much of an effect. A double-lumen dialysis catheter is inserted into the femoral or internal jugular vein and blood is filtered thorough a porous cellulose-based membrane that prevents removal of blood cells and large molecules. This process allows the return of the remaining blood to the body and only excess fluid is removed. Between 2 to 6 liters of fluid can be safely removed daily by this procedure and treatments over a week can help recovery from CHF.

In some patients with chronic CHF, implantation of a biventricular pacemaker is done when there is lack of coordination between the right and left ventricles due to scarring from myocardial infarction. In such cases, implantation of electrical leads in each ventricle resynchronizes cardiac contraction and boosts cardiac output. This procedure is described in Chapter 9. Implantable cardioverter-defibrillators (ICD) have been shown to be of benefit in prolonging the lives of patients with severe compensated CHF as the risk of sudden cardiac death due to ventricular fibrillation is high in such patients. Evolving guidelines for implantation of an ICD suggest that when the ejection fraction is 35 percent or less, there is a benefit in such treatment if the patient is more than 40 days out from a myocardial infarction.

Surgical Treatment for CHF

The majority of cases of CHF are treated with medications and dietary and fluid intake restrictions. Surgery is not often indicated to treat CHF. However, if there are valvular problems that are causing CHF, such as a leaking valve or aortic stenosis, this may be addressed by valve repair or replacement. In some cases of CHF, there may be areas of the heart that are ischemic and not receiving enough blood. Special tests done with metabolic agents and radiological isotopes may show that these areas of the heart may be suboptimally perfused with blood. Coronary bypass surgery may occasionally benefit the person by improving a severely decreased left ventricular ejection fraction. In such cases, revascularization with angioplasty or coronary bypass surgery may be useful to reestablish blood flow and improve the pumping action of the heart.

In patients with inherited hypertrophic cardiomyopathy, there is sometimes obstruction to blood flow from the left ventricle into the aorta. Surgery consisting of removal of part of the left ventricular septum is done using a microtome to shave off tissue to relieve obstruction. Alcohol injection into the septum to destroy excess muscle tissue can also be done in some cases to reduce the obstruction. These procedures are sometimes complicated by damage to the aortic valve during the surgical procedure, or by complete heart block due to damage to the conduction system of the heart.

In cases of severe CHF that is refractory to medical treatment and with a very low ejection fraction, heart transplantation is the only real option. A severe shortage of hearts is a serious limiting factor. As will be discussed in Chapter 10, artificial implanted hearts and heart assist devices are mainly bridging devices to a heart transplant.

END-OF-LIFE CARE

About 300,000 people die in the United States each year from CHF, and the number in Western Europe is probably higher. In the absence of heart transplantation, there is no other long-term treatment for patients with terminal heart failure when the heart is badly damaged. The cause of death is a gradual decline in cardiac output and blood pressure and slowing of the heartbeat so that the heart eventually stops and the patient succumbs. Palliative care is offered as an option and comfort measures provided to allow an easeful death.

A careful assessment needs to be made by not only the patient's cardiologist or internist, but also by a heart failure specialist, to be sure that little more can be done medically. A palliative care specialist, a social worker, as well as the family, should be included in all conferences about the patient. A realistic discussion should be had with the patient and a do-not-resuscitate order should be written. If the patient has an implanted cardioverter-defibrillator (ICD), a decision has to be made whether it should be turned off so that it is not activated if cardiac arrest occurs. Other decisions include whether patients should undergo dialysis, as kidney failure may set in when blood pressure declines. Use of other types of instrumentation and treatments should also be discussed (e.g., insertion of a balloon pump, a left ventricular assist device, gastric feeding tubes, and so forth). There is considerable controversy whether withholding of water and nutrients is ethically permissible with views that range from one extreme to the other. A voluntary decision to stop nutrition is permissible if the patient gives consent. An assessment about the patient's own decision-making capacity needs to be performed, as many patients are depressed and may not be in a condition to make this difficult decision. Depressed patients need psychiatric counseling and treatment.

In unconscious, mentally incompetent patients and in children, decision-making is an even more serious problem. The decision to terminate or withhold care can only be made after a joint consultation between the family and caregivers. The family should be warned that death may not occur for seven days or more after the patient stops being fed, and this may well be a painful ordeal for the family. To assuage feelings of guilt, the family members should be reassured they are making the right decision to withhold an unnatural prolongation of life, and that withholding unnecessary treatments only prevents the natural ending of life. Attention must also be paid to the family members as they may have severe emotional reactions to the impending death of a loved one. These issues complicate clinical decision making as they make it difficult to know what kinds of treatment are appropriate at the end of life.

Some patients may request euthanasia. Since euthanasia is illegal in the United States, the deliberate administration of drugs to a person with the intention to kill is not legally or ethically permissible. It is, however, permissible to give medications to relieve pain and suffering, and if death occurs as a result, this is considered a secondary effect that is permissible.

End-of-life care planning is a delicate issue that can divide families, pit them against caregivers, and cause emotional outbursts, and it takes extensive discussions and planning before being implemented. Since heart disease is a major cause of death, it consumes a great deal of resources that have to be used wisely. In terminally ill patients with congestive heart failure, we have to provide humane care and allow the comfortable ending of life so that patients do not undergo needless suffering.

6

Disorders of Cardiac Rhythm

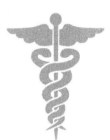

The heart is a human barometer that reacts to both the internal environment and to external changes. The internal environment, called the *milieu intérieur* by Claude Bernard (1813–1878), is the system in the body that maintains constant and stable conditions in temperature, acid–base balance, electrolyte levels, heart rate, blood pressure, and so forth. Multiple closed-loop systems with feedback regulation keep the body on an even keel. This condition is called *homeostasis*, a word coined by the great Harvard physiologist Walter Bradford Cannon (1871–1945). He also coined the term *fight or flight* response, to describe the body's response during an external threat when the body stokes up its defensive mechanisms, and pulse (heart) rate and blood pressure increase dramatically.

The heart reacts almost immediately to any disruption in internal and external changes. During a fever, the pulse rate increases due to the circulation of abnormal chemicals in the blood during an infection. If there is injury and blood loss, the pulse rate also increases while blood pressure decreases due to the loss in volume of circulating blood. We get pumped up when there is an external threat due to a discharge of adrenaline, and this leads to increases in heart rate and blood pressure. During such periods, the heart's rhythm may also become disrupted, with cardiac arrest occurring in rare cases.

The heart is a two-stage electromechanical pump where the atria contract first, followed a few milliseconds later by the ventricles. It normally beats regularly at about 60 to 70 beats per minute at rest and is capable of racing to as high as 250 beats per minute with maximal exercise. As described earlier, the heart has its own internal wiring system that keeps it beating regularly. Sometimes, this rhythm is disrupted due to disease of the heart muscle or problems within the conduction system itself.

The invention of the electrocardiogram (EKG) and the ability to record the heartbeat with long-term monitoring greatly simplified the diagnosis of heart rhythm abnormalities. Cardiac arrhythmias are divided into those that arise in the atria and those that arise in the ventricles. The normal rhythm of the heart is called *normal sinus rhythm* (NSR). In Figure 6.1, the first EKG strip shows NSR

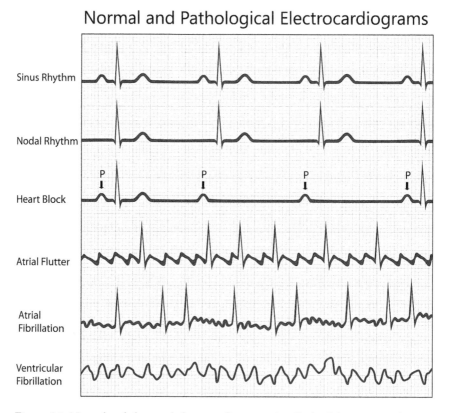

Normal and Pathological Electrocardiograms

Figure 6.1 Normal and abnormal electrocardiogram strips. Each of the six strips shows a single lead of an EKG. The first strip is normal sinus rhythm, and each of the other strips shows the labeled arrhythmia. © Alila07/Dreamstime.com.

and the succeeding five strips show a series of rhythms from five different patients with various arrhythmias. The second to the fifth EKG strips show atrial rhythms, where the configurations of the QRS complexes are similar to the QRS complex seen in NSR. The last strip shows ventricular fibrillation. This chapter will deal with the major rhythm abnormalities seen clinically. Detailed aspects of treatment for some of the specific arrhythmias, such as ventricular tachycardia and fibrillation, are dealt with in Chapter 11.

ATRIAL ARRHYTHMIAS

Atrial Premature Beats

The normal heart can occasionally throw off extra beats called atrial premature beats (APB). These beats are extremely common and occur frequently, especially with advancing age. Such extra beats appear very similar to normal beats on the EKG with some variation in the configuration of the P waves. They do not cause problems even when they occur in short bursts of 8 to 10 beats at a time, when they are called *supraventricular tachycardia* (SVT). No treatment is necessary, and the patient can be reassured that the heart is normal if this is the only finding. The person may be unaware of its occurrence, but occasionally, there is a feeling of a "flip-flop" in the heart or the patient may say he has an unpleasant gulping feeling in the chest. No treatment needs to be given, though a beta-blocking agent may help if there is chest discomfort from a sensation of flip-flops and short bursts of SVT.

Atrial Tachycardia (Supraventricular Tachycardia)

When APBs occur in repetitive salvoes, as described, this is called paroxysmal atrial tachycardia (PAT) or supraventricular tachycardia (SVT). This type of rhythm disturbance needs treatment if it is of prolonged duration or causing symptoms. Patients complain of a furious and rapid thumping in the chest that is frightening if the arrhythmia is sustained for several minutes or hours. Some people report they feel a sensation characterized as "my heart is going to jump out of my mouth." This sensation is frightening, especially if the heart rate is very fast. Sometimes, shortness of breath and chest tightness occurs. Since blood pressure may decline rapidly during SVT, dizziness and fainting occur in some people. Typically the rate is 180–220 beats per minute and regular, with a sudden onset and offset of which the person is aware. Often the diagnosis can be made just by the description of symptoms, and an EKG done during an episode of SVT will confirm this diagnosis.

This rhythm abnormality can be caused by some congenital abnormalities, thyroid hyperactivity, and excessive use of caffeine, alcohol, sugar, or illegal drugs, such as cocaine and amphetamines. Acute psychological stress can also cause SVT. Excessive fatigue combined with insomnia or sleep deprivation lowers the threshold for this arrhythmia, especially when acute psychological stress is an additional provoking factor.

The rhythm can arise from an ectopic focus in the atria, causing the heart to beat very rapidly. Another variety results from abnormal pathways in the conduction system. Some people are born with extra electrical pathways around the AV node that are called *accessory pathways* or *bypass tracts*. These extra bundles of conductive tissue are present at birth and generally are supposed to shut down as the heart matures. However, in some people these bypass tracts persist well into adolescence and adulthood.

An atrial premature beat traveling into the ventricles through the normal atrioventricular (AV) node first activates the ventricles and then makes a U-turn and reenters the node through an abnormal pathway that bypasses the AV node. The impulse then reenters the atria and activates them. The electrical impulse does not stop there, but circulates back into the ventricles through the AV node. This process is repeated at rates of 200 to 500 beats per minute so that a circulating rhythm is set up, making the heart beat very fast. Sometimes, the tract is not near the AV node, but elsewhere in the heart, connecting the junction between the atria and the ventricles. This abnormal rhythm is called a *reentrant arrhythmia*, occurring through an accessory pathway.

Initial treatment of SVT consists of applying firm pressure with two fingers to the neck over the upper part of the carotid artery for 30 seconds. This process increases vagal nerve stimulation to the heart and can terminate SVT. Medications such as adenosine and calcium channel blockers are also used to terminate SVT. Electrophysiologic testing using electrical intracardiac catheters can identify the presence of accessory pathways and locate them with precision. In such cases, the best way to treat SVT is to perform radiofrequency ablation of the accessory pathway through the catheter. This procedure is the preferred treatment, especially in young subjects, as it is often curative, and long-term drug treatment can be avoided.

Atrial Fibrillation

Atrial fibrillation (AF) is an important cardiac disorder that makes the heart beat irregularly. In Figure 6.1 it can be seen on the fifth EKG strip, where the fine irregular baseline is made up of "f," or fibrillation, waves. It is one of the most commonly occurring of important cardiac arrhythmias, and it increases in incidence with age. Over 2 million people in the United States alone suffer from AF. During AF, there is irregular uncoordinated activity of the atria that wriggles and writhes at 400–600 times a minute. The AV node serves as a gate blocking many of the impulses, so that only about half or less of these beats get through to the ventricles.

In this scenario, because pumping action of the atria is lost, cardiac output can decline by as much as 25–30 percent in AF. It is a complex arrhythmia, as there are many causes and the presence of AF on an EKG is only a symptom of some other underlying disorder. Hence, treatment needs to take into consideration the underlying condition that triggered AF in the first place.

There are three groups of causal factors associated with AF. In the first group, the atria are normal, but there are transient risk factors that stimulate the atria, provoking AF as a one-time event or one that recurs only infrequently. Extrinsic causes such as caffeine, alcohol, and drugs such as cocaine can provoke AF, as can thyroid overactivity. Other transient factors include temporary states that cause low oxygenation (*hypoxia*) due to conditions such as pneumonia, congestive heart failure, chronic lung disease, and pulmonary embolism. It can also occur during surgery or postoperatively due to changes in oxygenation during and following surgical anesthesia. When AF occurs in these situations, it is rapid, with rates of 130–220 beats per minute. The arrhythmia, once treated, does not tend to recur, as it is essentially secondary to a transient external trigger. Therefore, extensive cardiac testing and ongoing treatment with medications is often unnecessary.

A second group of underlying causes relates to some anatomical problem that resides in the heart and the arrhythmia is secondary to heart disease. Examples of this group are sick sinus syndrome, abnormal bypass tracts, distention and scarring of the atria in rheumatic heart disease, valvular heart disease, atrial infarction, and pericarditis. This kind of AF becomes recurrent or permanent. In sick sinus syndrome, the conduction system as a whole slows down due to the aging process. The sinoatrial node fails to beat normally and may do so only at rates of 20–40 beats per minute. The atrioventricular node often does not conduct impulses to the ventricles normally, producing pauses in the EKG for 10 seconds or more and resulting in a condition called *heart block*. The patient may feel weak and pass out if heart block results in several seconds of absent electrical and mechanical action called *asystole*. The treatment here is implantation of a permanent electronic pacemaker to take over the function of the natural cardiac pacemaker. This condition is often referred to as *sick sinus syndrome*. Treatment is thus not just for the AF itself, but also for the underlying cause of AF, due to a sick conduction system.

A third type of arrhythmia is called *lone atrial fibrillation*. In this condition, AF occurs with no apparent known cause. The condition is very resistant to treatment and repeated attempts to revert it to sinus rhythm often fail. This rhythm disturbance is difficult to treat with medicines, and cardioversion with electrical energy is often unsuccessful. One option is to leave the patient in AF with an anticoagulant to prevent clot formation and embolism that can lead to a stroke. However, today a good option is electrophysiologic catheter ablation to terminate AF.

Symptoms may be absent in many cases where the rate in AF is moderate and the condition is often only discovered during a routine office visit. However, if the onset is sudden, and the rate very rapid, the person will experience alarming palpitations and may feel weak, dizzy, and short of breath. Chest pain is not common. In fact, most people with AF are completely unaware they have this arrhythmia, and it is discovered only during a routine EKG in a doctor's office or on admission to hospital for other reasons. If AF is due to thyroid overactivity, there will be symptoms of tremor, sweating, weight loss, and so forth. All patients with AF should have a thyroid hormone screening test, as this condition is very treatable. The initial diagnosis of AF is made by an EKG recording. However, a search must be made for an underlying cause: echocardiography to rule out heart muscle and valve disease, as well as electrophysiologic testing, if appropriate.

Treatment depends on the underlying cause. Offending causes such as alcohol, caffeine, drugs, and stimulants should be removed. Hypoxia needs to be corrected with oxygen, either temporarily or with continuous flow. Thyroid disease needs to be treated with appropriate medications and once this is done, the arrhythmia will subside. If there is sick sinus syndrome due to conduction system disease, a permanent pacemaker needs to be installed to correct the conduction abnormality.

A variety of drugs have been used to treat AF, including disopyramide, flecainide, amiodarone, dronedarone, propafenone, sotalol, and dofetilide. Many of these drugs may have serious side effects and treatment should be carefully monitored to check for side effects. Cardioversion with electricity terminates AF immediately, unless it is long-standing, in which case AF recurs almost immediately or shortly after following cardioversion.

In 1987, James Cox, a surgeon at Barnes Hospital in St. Louis, Missouri, introduced the *maze procedure* to terminate AF. This procedure requires open chest surgery and consists of making incisions into both atria to prevent reentry of the fibrillation waves, thus terminating AF. More recently, electrical ablation of the areas around the openings of four pulmonary veins into the left atrium has been found to terminate AF. This procedure is done with a catheter threaded through the groin and does not require chest surgery. Short bursts of radiofrequency waves eliminate trigger points around the pulmonary veins, preventing reentry of AF waves and terminating the arrhythmia.

The most feared complication in AF is the release of clots from the atria into the arterial circulation that can travel to the brain and cause a stroke. Clots can also enter the coronary artery and cause a myocardial infarction. Similarly, they may enter a limb artery and cause ischemia of an arm or leg. Clots form in the atria due to stasis of blood as it swirls in these chambers, and the atria do not contract to expel blood efficiently into the ventricles. Thus, anticoagulation, with a drug like warfarin (Coumadin), needs to be performed to prevent blood from clotting easily. Anticoagulation is also done before cardioversion, otherwise clots that adhere to the walls of the atria may be discharged into the circulation and cause embolic complications. In 2010, the Food and Drug Administration approved dabigatran (Pradaxa) for anticoagulation in AF. For immediate treatment to prevent clot formation in AF, the intravenous or subcutaneously administered medication heparin is used as it acts rapidly, within hours. It is given regularly, while an oral anticoagulant is also started because the latter only begins to take effect after several days. Heparin is therefore used intravenously to provide prophylaxis before the oral drug takes effect.

In patients who undergo cardioversion or an electrophysiologic procedure for its termination, the anticoagulant is continued for at least four weeks after the procedure as AF may relapse. If sinus rhythm is maintained, anticoagulation is terminated, as complications from bleeding are a serious problem, and even death may occur, especially in older patients.

Atrial Flutter

Atrial flutter (AFL) was first described in 1920 by Sir Thomas Lewis (1881–1945), the great British cardiologist who was the first to use the EKG extensively to diagnose arrhythmias. AFL causes a regular and very characteristic *sawtooth* pattern on the EKG occurring about 300 times a minute. This sawtooth pattern is due to "F" waves, as seen in Figure 6.1 in the fourth EKG strip. Due to the presence of a condition called atrioventricular (AV) block (occurring even in normal hearts), not all the atrial impulses get through to the ventricles when the atria beat at very fast rates of 300 times a minute or more. In such cases, due to AV block, the ventricle responds at exactly half or one-third of the atrial rate, as only one out of two or one out of three atrial impulses makes it to the ventricles. Therefore, if the atrial rate is 300 beats per minute, the ventricle responds at either 150 or 100 beats per minute, depending on the degree of AV block. In the

EKG strip in Figure 6.1, proceeding from left to right, there is variable block with 4:1, 2:1, and 3:1 AV block, resulting in a proportionally varying heart rate. This phenomenon is a protective device to prevent the ventricles from beating too rapidly, as very fast rates makes the heart inefficient. Cardiac output decreases rather than increases at very high rates.

Unlike the situation in AF, clots typically do not form in the heart, as there are regular contractions of the atria. However, AFL may degenerate into AF or there may be periods of fibrillation along with flutter, increasing the possibility of clot formation inside the atria. It is customary, therefore, to use anticoagulation in AFL, as one cannot be sure that fibrillation is not concomitantly present.

Patients with AFL often do not know they have the rhythm, as it does not cause palpitations in many cases. Sometimes, there is a sensation of fluttering in the chest. If conduction to the ventricles is not blocked at the level of the AV node, the heart may beat at 300 beats per minute, resulting in a sensation of alarming palpitations, and the person may feel dizzy or faint.

Treatment is the same as for AF with the same group of drugs. Unlike AF, which requires higher doses of electricity, AFL is very easily reverted with lower doses during cardioversion, and sometimes with the application of as little as five joules of energy. Anticoagulation guidelines for cardioversion are similar to those for AF.

Wolf-Parkinson-White Syndrome

Normally, an electrical impulse travels from the right atrium down the atrio-ventricular (AV) node to the ventricles. The AV node controls the number of impulses that can get into the ventricles if there is a very high rate of firing of an abnormal focus in the atria. In Wolf-Parkinson-White (WPW) syndrome, there is an abnormal connection between the atria and the ventricles called the Bundle of Kent that bypasses the AV node and connects the atria directly with the ventricles. In this condition, the bundle is situated at the sides of the heart, well away from the AV node. This allows an atrial premature beat to conduct very rapidly into the ventricle through this abnormal pathway and then travel backward through the normal conduction system and reenter the atria through the AV node. The impulse can then repeat the process, entering the ventricles again through the Bundle of Kent and repeating this process hundreds of times a minute, to produce heart rates of 300–400 beats per minute. The abnormal rhythms seen may be supraventricular tachycardia or atrial fibrillation.

This situation can be dangerous and lead to cardiac arrest from ventricular fibrillation and sudden death in rare instances. When WPW is at slower rates, it can be treated with medications until definitive treatment with electrical ablation can be done. However, if it results in ultra-rapid heart rates, this is a true medical emergency as cardiac arrest can follow. In this situation, the patient needs to be immediately electrically cardioverted to avoid cardiac arrest from ventricular fibrillation.

Roughly 1 in 1,000 people have WPW syndrome, and it is associated with an abnormal gene in some people. The patient often feels palpitations from early childhood onward. The EKG is diagnostic as it shows a characteristic *delta wave* at the beginning of the QRS complex that leads to an unmistakable slurring of the upstroke of the R wave. The preferred treatment is to perform radiofrequency ablation of the bypass tract. Since the subjects are young, this procedure, if suc-cessful, is curative and avoids the necessity for unpleasant drug treatment for a lifetime.

Nodal (Junctional) Rhythm

Nodal or junctional rhythm refers to a rhythm arising from the region of the atrioventricular (AV) node. This rhythm occurs when the sinus node fails to discharge or does so at a very slow rate. Figure 6.1 shows this rhythm in the second strip from the top. The rhythm is recognizable when there is no P-wave visible. Sometimes there is an inverted P-wave or a P-wave that follows the QRS-complex. This situation arises when the sinus node is diseased (*sick sinus syn-drome*) or when there is a condition that allows the AV node to beat faster than the sinus node. The latter condition sometimes occurs spontaneously during slow heart rates during sleep, in inferior myocardial infarction, when there is digitalis toxicity, or when provoked by an atrial premature beat that engages in reentry through the AV node. The last condition is referred to as *junctional tachycardia,* as already discussed above. The rate of nodal or junctional rhythm is usually around 40–60 beats per minute. In accelerated junctional rhythm (junctional tachycar-dia), the rates are more rapid and over 100 beats per minute.

Nodal rhythm when it occurs at a slow rate is usually not a problem in itself. If it occurs during sleep, no treatment is necessary. If it occurs during inferior myo-cardial infarction, and the heart rate is very low, an artificial pacemaker may be needed to maintain a normal heart rate. The underlying cause has to be treated if the rate is rapid and the patient is symptomatic as discussed for supraventricular tachycardia.

Heart Block

The term *heart block,* as discussed previously, does not refer to a physical block, but an *electrical* block that prevents normal sinus beats from traversing the AV node and traveling to the ventricles. This rhythm is seen in Figure 6.1 in the third strip from the top. The block occurs because the AV node fails to conduct the sinus P-wave properly. The strip shows 4 P-waves, of which the first and fourth P-waves conduct normally, but the second and the third P-waves do not conduct through the AV node. This condition may occur due to intrinsic disease of the AV node or due to the action of drugs such as digitalis glycosides and calcium channel blocking agents on the AV node.

In Lev-Lenègre disease, independently described by Maurice Lev and Jean Lenègre, there is fibrosis of the conduction system, and the patient develops a very slow pulse and faints when the heart rate decreases to about 30 beats per minute. The treatment is to insert a temporary pacemaker if the condition is deemed to be due to a transient cause. However, if the condition persists, a permanent pacemaker should be implanted.

VENTRICULAR ARRHYTHMIAS

Ventricular Premature Beats

As the heart ages, it gives off occasional extra beats called ventricular premature beats (VPB), arising spontaneously from the heart muscle. It is called *premature* because the beat occurs earlier than the expected sinus beat. Sometimes VPBs occur in couplets or triplets. Generally, VPBs are benign and do not produce any problems other than the sensation of a missed beat. The person actually does not feel the extra beat, but the next normal beat that is expected will not occur, and hence there is an abnormally long pause until a normal beat occurs. The patient therefore reports that he has experienced a skipped beat. No treatment is necessary, but troublesome symptoms can be treated with a beta-adrenergic blocker, such as propranolol or metoprolol.

Ventricular Tachycardia

Ventricular tachycardia (VT) is a repetitive firing of the ventricles at rates that may range from 100 to 400 or so. In many cases, VT may degenerate into ventricular fibrillation (VF). The causes include spontaneous activity of the ventricles with no known heart disease, during a myocardial infarction (MI), or abnormal impulses arising from the edges of a healed scar following healing from an MI. If the rate is fast, blood pressure may decline and VT needs to be terminated quickly. In the case of VT occurring in the setting of an MI, or after recovery from an MI, there is the possibility that cardiac arrest may occur due to ventricular fibrillation. Such a scenario requires immediate treatment with intravenous amiodarone or procainamide, or with electrical cardioversion.

Sometimes, pulseless VT occurs, where the rate is rapid and there is really no cardiac output. This situation rapidly progresses to VF with unconsciousness occurring, and this situation requires immediate defibrillation as it constitutes an emergency.

The diagnosis is made by an EKG or during telemetry monitoring of the EKG in the hospital setting. Treatment with medications as noted above is indicated; however, in most cases today, a cardioverter-defibrillator is implanted in patients deemed at high risk for cardiac arrest. In some cases, when a reentrant pathway for VT can be identified, radiofrequency ablation can be done to terminate the condition permanently.

A special variety of VT is called *torsades de pointes* ("twisting around a point"). It has a characteristic appearance on an EKG that is diagnostic due to a very recognizable waxing and waning of the QRS complex. Torsades is generally caused by drugs such as lithium, quinidine, sotalol, procainamide, and phenothiazines that prolong the QT interval of the EKG. There is a risk that *torsades* can progress to VF and death.

Treatment consists of withdrawing the offending agent and administration of magnesium sulfate. If cardiac arrest is imminent, defibrillation is performed, as delivery of synchronized shock is not possible due to extreme variations in the QRS complex.

Accelerated Idioventricular Rhythm

Accelerated idioventricular rhythm (AIVR) is similar to VT, but at a rate of 100 beats per minute or less. The ventricular rate is higher that the intrinsic rate of the ventricles of about 20-40 beats per minute. This rhythm is seen during recovery from MI, digitalis toxicity, and cardiomyopathy. Though it is a slower version of ventricular tachycardia, it is generally benign and does not progress to cardiac arrest. Treatment of the underlying cause is sufficient, with no specific therapy directed at AIVR.

Ventricular Fibrillation

Ventricular fibrillation (VF) is the chaotic depolarization of the ventricular myocardium resulting in cardiac arrest and sudden death if untreated. In the Western world, sudden death from VF is the single most important cause of death. This disorder can occur in structurally normal hearts, or in hearts that have been damaged by myocarditis, cardiomyopathy, or myocardial infarction. However, by far and away, the commonest cause of VF is coronary artery disease.

The specifics of the origins of VF and its treatment are dealt with in detail in Chapter 11, "Cardiac Arrest and Resuscitation." One of the challenges for researchers working on VF is to discover ways to identify future victims of this deadly arrhythmia. A major advance in the last 50 years is the discovery that beta-adrenergic blockers reduce the incidence of sudden death after myocardial infarction.

SUMMARY

The heart can generate abnormal rhythms originating in the atria or the ventricles. Atrial arrhythmias are generally benign and not life-threatening. However, in some instances, atrial arrhythmias can cause symptoms such as fainting and also lead to cardiac arrest when they occur at ultra-rapid rates. Another feared complication is the discharge of clots from the left atrium in atrial fibrillation, leading to cerebrovascular strokes.

Ventricular arrhythmias are generally more serious and life-threatening as in the case of rapid ventricular tachycardia and VF. The most common cause of VF is coronary artery disease. At present, it is not possible to predict VF with any accuracy, and much research is directed at trying to identify future victims of this fatal arrhythmia.

7

Congenital Heart Disease

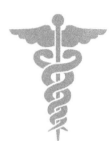

Congenital heart disease (CHD) refers to a group of cardiac abnormalities that occur due to faulty development of the heart during fetal life. Such disorders result from both genetic predisposition and environmental factors. Prenatal risk factors include exposure of the parents to certain biological hazards such as drugs, chemicals, and radiation that damage the genetic material in ova and sperm. This type of heart disease is the leading cause of death in newborn infants in most Western countries. In the United States, out of a population of 315 million, there are about 1 million people living with CHD presently. These disorders are present at birth, affecting about 1 out of 124 infants. Because of the vast variety of genetic defects that occur in humans, only the most common major cardiac abnormalities and other rare, but important, disorders will be described.

In most cases, the defects are in the heart itself, and in others, they are located outside the heart in the great vessels attached in proximity to the heart. In a minority of patients, defects may occur in both the heart and in the great vessels. Three groups of CHD can be identified by the way they present clinically: (1) those that cause problems at birth or in early life; (2) those that cause problems later in adolescence and in adulthood; and (3) functional problems that cannot be seen anatomically, but that can cause arrhythmias or death due to electrical derangements.

CONGENITAL HEART DEFECTS PRESENTING IN EARLY LIFE

The development of the human heart is quite an extraordinary process. The heart starts as a tubular structure in the fetus, begins to beat spontaneously only three weeks after conception, and initially mirrors the mother's heartbeat of 70 to 80 beats per minute. As it grows, the heart rate increases to about 170 beats per minute by the second month and decelerates to about 140 at the time of birth. The tubular progenitor to the heart loops and folds in on itself to form a common atrium and a common ventricle like a fish heart. It then separates into three and then into a total of four chambers with the development of muscular walls dividing the atria and the ventricles. Throughout this process, the valves also begin to form to control the flow of blood that is produced in the bone marrow and finds its way into the heart through newly formed blood vessels.

This complicated process is controlled by a series of genes that guides the formation of each of the anatomical components of the heart. During this complex process, any number of things can go wrong, including malformations of the chambers, the separations between them, the valves, and the conduction system. Almost 10 percent of people suffer embryonic malformations in one or more of these structures and are subsequently born with heart defects. Such defects are the commonest immediate cause of death following delivery. In fact, many fetuses with serious congenital cardiac defects abort spontaneously as the wisdom of the body seems to realize that these malformations make survival impossible.

Some congenital heart defects such as *Fallot's tetralogy* or *transposition of the great vessels* are very serious, and they are due to anatomical malformations of the major blood vessels attached to the heart. Such defects are identified at birth or in very early infancy and childhood. These abnormalities are often so severe that they cause immediate problems following birth, and it is quite obvious that something is amiss with the cardiovascular system. In some cases, failure to thrive leads to a doctor's visit for a definitive diagnosis and treatment.

HEART DEFECTS EMERGING LATER IN LIFE

Some genetic defects are present at birth, but they do not produce any structural alterations at birth because they do not immediately impair cardiac pumping action. However, as the child grows, the abnormality leads to structural changes in cardiac structure and function due to a continued strain on heart function. Thus, these defects emerge only much later in life to impair cardiac function. The heart appears to be apparently normal at birth and in early life because no structural changes are observed on a cursory physical examination or on X-rays.

Very small atrial septal defects may be completely overlooked until the person is in the fourth and fifth decades of life. Small ventricular septal defects may also be overlooked until adolescence and adulthood. Another prominent example is *hypertrophic cardiomyopathy* (HCM), where heart muscle thickens, causing obstruction to blood flow from the left ventricle. The person seems normal in early life, but symptoms develop usually only in adulthood as the heart muscle thickens progressively and causes obstructive symptoms. In the case of HCM, the person is also susceptible to sudden death from cardiac arrest. Death may occur on the football field, as happens occasionally in school and college sports. The abnormality is then discovered only on autopsy.

The diagnosis is made during a routine office visit when the doctor hears a heart murmur. In some cases, the baby or child demonstrates failure to thrive, or becomes short of breath or has frequent respiratory infections. Often, the diagnosis comes as a shock to a parent or the patient himself. The question arises: "If this was a congenital defect, why was it not discovered at birth?" The reason is that the heart defect was simply missed at birth, or that children have benign murmurs so often that it was not considered pathological until the child developed symptoms that deserved medical attention.

Because some structural defects resolve spontaneously with growth, it is advisable to wait further development before performing invasive diagnostic tests and surgery. This is the case in small atrial and ventricular septal defects, where spontaneous closure may occur.

DISORDERS CAUSING FUNCTIONAL ABNORMALITIES

Another group of abnormalities are functional in nature and not anatomical, so that the heart seems structurally normal on external examination. These disorders most often cause alterations in the electrical functions of the heart. Many of these functional disorders lead to cardiac arrhythmias, such as atrial tachycardia or ventricular fibrillation, that cause sudden death at a young age. In the case of abnormal bypass tracts in the heart, the changes are in the conduction system of the heart and hardly visible extra pathways exist in between the atria and ventricles. These pathways lead to a phenomenon called *preexcitation* that causes atrial arrhythmias in many cases. Since an atrial impulse can go down the extra pathway, it arrives in the ventricles earlier than normal and excites the ventricles prematurely. Hence, the name *preexcitation syndrome* is given to these arrhythmias. These rhythm disturbances may be present in childhood, but in many cases they become apparent only in adolescence and early adulthood. Microscopic examination during autopsy will reveal the location of these abnormal tracts. Many atrial tachycardias such as the Lown-Ganong-Levine syndrome and the Wolff-Parkinson-White syndrome are caused by abnormal intracardiac bypass tracts that are present from birth. Such arrhythmias are collectively called *preexcitation syndromes*. In such cases, symptoms are self-limited and require only intermittent treatment when an atrial tachycardia breaks out.

Other important examples of functional disorders are the long QT interval syndrome (LQTS), Jervell-Lange-Nielsen syndrome, and Romano-Ward syndrome, all of which can lead to sudden death from cardiac arrest in adolescence. The Brugada syndrome was identified in 1992 by the Spanish cardiologists Pedro and Josep Brugada as a genetic abnormality that leads to sudden death in young men.

These abnormalities are genetically transmitted and are due to chromosomal mutations that eventually result in abnormal repolarization of the ventricles. Over a dozen genetic abnormalities have been identified in LQTS alone. Many of these functional abnormalities were clearly recognized only in the last few decades, and tools for precise genetic diagnosis were not available until recently. New methods for diagnosis and treatment using genetic manipulations are still being developed for these diseases. Results from these new treatments have yet to be evaluated fully, as the experience with such treatments is still very limited.

While genetic testing is now more widely available, the most difficult clinical problem with such genetic abnormalities is how to counsel patients. Genetic counseling services are still not as widely available as the ability to test for genetic abnormalities. What a person should do when a genetic test shows a mutation that could cause problems years down the line is still an open question.

CAUSES OF CONGENITAL HEART DISEASE

The actual causes of many congenital heart diseases are often unknown. However, there are at least four broad categories of causes that can sometimes be identified accurately: genetic, infections (and other diseases), toxins, and radiation exposure.

Genetic Causes

There are several chromosomal and genetic abnormalities that are associated with CHD. Chromosomes are microscopic structures containing all of an individual's genetic information that live in the nucleus of every cell, except for red blood cells, as these cells lack a nucleus. The chromosomes are composed of various proteins and deoxyribonucleic acid (DNA) that contains the entire genetic code of an individual in every cell. The DNA contains *codes* that control specific functions of that particular cell. Through a process known as *gene expression*, only selected portions of the DNA codes are expressed. Thus, only the DNA necessary for the functioning of the brain is expressed in brain cells and only the material needed for functioning of heart muscle is expressed in the myocardium. However, all of the genetic material needed for a brain cell or any other type of cell is also contained within the myocardial cell nucleus.

In humans, there are about 25,000 genes contained in 46 chromosomes that come in 23 pairs in every cell. In each pair, one chromosome comes from the father and the other from the mother. Therefore, half the chromosomes in each cell come from the father and the other half from the mother. One pair is the *sex chromosome*, which is designated XX in females and XY in males. In males, there is one X chromosome from the mother and a shorter Y chromosome from the father. Besides the sex chromosomes, the other 22 pairs are called *autosomal chromosomes* as they control nonsexual functions of the body. There are collections of specific proteins on a chromosome that are called *genes*, which are the molecular units of heredity.

When cells divide, the pairs of chromosomes separate and duplicate themselves to form two sister chromosomes. Chromosomes in a pair may also exchange material with the adjoining chromosome while undergoing division. In this rearrangement, often nothing goes wrong. However, during such rearrangements, sometimes a piece of genetic material fragments and breaks off and thus becomes lost in the interior of the cell. This loss of genetic material is called a *deletion*. In other cases, a piece of one chromosome attaches to the wrong chromosome during cell division and this is called a *translocation*. Rarely, an entire chromosome winds up in a sister cell so that there are three chromosomes instead of only a pair (e.g., in *Trisomy 21* or *Down syndrome*). These abnormal changes are collectively called *mutations*. Such mutations are commoner when a mother conceives for the first time after the age of 35, when the father is in an older age group, or when the reproductive cells are exposed to ionizing radiation.

Abnormalities may be passed from parents to children when deletions, translocations, or extra chromosomes occur during the division of sex chromosomes.

When fetal cells divide, there is also a chance that genetic mistakes may occur, though the parents may be normal. Fetal abnormalities can sometimes be detected before birth. Amniocentesis is a procedure done by removing amniotic fluid from the womb when a woman is pregnant. Testing of the cells found floating in the amniotic fluid can reveal chromosomal abnormalities, thus allowing a diagnosis to be made. Chromosomal analysis done on cells obtained from other types of cells, such as from the inside of the cheek, can also help diagnose genetic abnormalities in adults.

The most commonly known example of a genetic cause of congenital heart disease is that of Down syndrome, in which there is a presence of all or part of an extra chromosome 21. Therefore, this condition is called *Trisomy 21*, and it leads to both physical and cognitive developmental impairment. Children are recognizable by their facial features, such as a round face, a small chin, slanting eyes, an oversized tongue, a short stature, and mental impairment. Some children also have a cardiac defect, such as a ventricular septal defect. There are other kinds of chromosomal defects (e.g., Trisomy 13 and 18) that are also associated with CHD and much more severe mental impairment than is seen with Trisomy 21.

In *Turner syndrome* there is only an X chromosome; the other X or Y chromosome is missing and the genotype is called XO. The person is female in appearance with characteristically recognizable features such as a low stature, webbed neck, a flat chest with widely spaced nipples, and amenorrhea. About 45 percent of Turner syndrome patients have cardiovascular abnormalities such as aortic stenosis and a narrowing of the aorta close to the heart, called *coarctation*. In most cases, the parents are unaware the child with either Down or Turner syndrome has a cardiac defect, as the diagnosis may not be obvious at the time of birth. An abnormality is discovered in later childhood or adolescence when facial and physical features are better developed and a murmur is heard.

Infections and Other Diseases

Most of the major organs are formed in the first three months of fetal life. Therefore, exposure of the fetus to any infection or toxin when the organs are being actively formed may cause malformation of the heart and other organs. The best-known infection that causes CHD is *rubella*, or German measles. The virus crosses the placenta into the fetus and causes serious heart, brain, and eye damage, as well as deafness. The most common heart defect in *rubella* is *patent ductus arteriosus*. Protection can be obtained with rubella vaccine, as this is the best measure a woman can take against developing an infection that may affect her baby.

Other viruses and infections that can cause congenital malformations affecting the heart and other organs are herpes, cytomegalovirus, measles, human immunodeficiency virus (HIV), and toxoplasmosis. Diseases such as diabetes, lupus, and phenylketonuria (PKU) interfere with normal fetal development, especially in the first trimester of pregnancy. These conditions are also associated with several congenital heart malformations.

Drugs and Chemicals

Drugs and chemicals that cause fetal abnormalities are said to be *teratogenic*. A wide variety of drugs can cause congenital heart defects. A teratogenic effect from a drug is most likely to occur in the first three months of pregnancy, as this is when organs are being formed in the fetus. Alcohol crosses the placenta and can affect the fetus. Excessive use of alcohol causes *fetal alcohol syndrome*, which results in mental and structural damage to the brain and the heart as well as the eyes and other internal organs. Ventricular septal defects, followed by atrial septal defects, are the most common heart abnormalities due to alcohol toxicity.

Certain medications such as thalidomide, lithium, and hydantoin are well known to have teratogenic effects on the heart. Many other drugs are contra-indicated in pregnancy and several come with a warning that they may affect the fetus. Families should be counseled in cases where the fetus may have been exposed to drugs or toxins, as the baby may be born with abnormalities. Parents may have to make a difficult choice as to whether they wish to risk this outcome and have the baby, or to abort the fetus.

Radiation

During a nuclear explosion or a meltdown, about 200 or more radioactive isotopes are released. The effects of such radiation were studied on survivors of the atomic bombing of Hiroshima and Nagasaki in 1945 and the Chernobyl disaster in 1986. In such disasters, the gonads are radiated directly so that reproductive cells become damaged by intense radiation. Studies showed not only an increase in cancers of many organs and leukemia, but also an increase in birth defects in children born to the survivors. Radiation causes both genetic mutation and fractionation of chromosomes. The result is multiple birth defects including cleft palate, mental deficiency, neurological abnormalities, and defects in the limbs and internal organs. Down syndrome and cardiac defects also occurred in children born to the victims of the atomic bomb blasts and the Chernobyl disaster.

Repeated exposure to X-rays may damage sperm and ova, and so the testes and ovaries need to be protected using lead shields over the lower part of the body during radiological procedures. Women in the reproductive age group should avoid exposure to radiation if they are planning to have children. Pregnant women should not receive X-rays unless absolutely necessary as radiation may affect the fetus, especially in the first trimester. Younger women should also not engage in work where there is a possibility of high radiation exposure such as in some hospital areas and in nuclear power plants.

TYPES OF CONGENITAL HEART DISEASE

Congenital heart disease can affect the chambers of the heart, the septa separating the chambers, the valves, the great vessels, and the arteries and veins that feed the heart or are connected with it. Nonstructural diseases include genetic and electrical defects that may not be visible by tests such as echocardiography early on in life. The most common type of CHD results from the incomplete development of internal cardiac structures leading to abnormal connections between two or more of the cardiac chambers. These defects are colloquially called *holes in the heart*. Blood is shunted between the chambers in either direction due to pressure differences in the chambers.

Structural heart defects are classified clinically as being either *cyanotic* or *non-cyanotic heart disease*. (Cyanosis is a term derived from the color *cyan*, which is a bluish color similar to that seen in venous blood.) Arterial blood is red and venous blood has a dark purple-blue color so that when venous blood enters the arterial system, arterial blood becomes darker and in a light-skinned person, the lips and fingertips turn blue. The clinical classification of cyanotic and non-cyanotic heart disease is based on whether there is mixing of arterial blood with venous blood. Cyanosis occurs only when venous blood from the right side of the heart or pulmonary artery enters the left heart circulation and mixes with arterial blood.

If a connection exists between the left side and the right side of the heart (as in a ventricular septal defect), arterial blood from the left ventricle is injected into venous blood in the right ventricle and there is no cyanosis. Shunting of blood occurs from the arterial side to the venous side and into the pulmonary circulation because the pressure in the left heart is higher than in the right heart.

Arterial blood turns blue when blood from the right side of the heart is shunted to the left side due to reversals in pressure through an atrial or ventricular septal defect or though some other channel. This phenomenon is called *shunt reversal* and it occurs when the blood pressure in the pulmonary circulation exceeds the pressure in the systemic circulation. Though the pressure in the left heart system is normally higher than in the right heart system, this situation changes after many years of increased flow from the left side to the right side of the heart. After years of coping with higher blood volumes and pressures than normal, the low-pressure pulmonary vascular bed becomes damaged as it suffers the effects of higher and higher blood pressure over many years. The pulmonary vascular bed becomes thickened and resistance increases due to a long-standing and excessive hemodynamic stress over many years. This process causes the blood pressure in the pulmonary arteries to increase and leads to pulmonary vascular obstructive disease. The condition is called *pulmonary hypertension*, which is an irreversible physiological state. Eventually, the pulmonary artery pressure exceeds the pressure in the left ventricle and the left atrium. Because the pressure in the right side of the heart is now higher than the left side, blood is now pumped from the right atrium to the left atrium (in the case of atrial septal defect) or from the right ventricle to the left side. This situation is called *shunt reversal* or *right-to-left shunting* and results in venous blood being pumped into the arterial system. Cyanosis results when a large amount of venous blood is shunted into the arterial system following the reversal of flow from the venous to the arterial side.

The mixture of arterial and venous blood results in a lowering of the oxygen saturation from 100 percent in arterial blood to about 70 percent or less. The blood also looks more blue than red, from whence we get the term *blue baby*. In simple terms, when there is cyanosis, it means that the condition has progressed to an advanced stage and complex pressure changes have already occurred over many years to cause *pulmonary hypertension*, resulting in reversal of blood flow from the right heart to the left heart. In this advanced stage of shunt reversal, the risk for complications and death during surgical correction of the septal defect is increased and death may occur. An operation is not only risky but may not succeed in correcting the problem as pulmonary hypertension cannot be reversed.

Over time, because of the abnormally high pressure in the right heart system, the person becomes short of breath and has limited exercise capacity, and congestive heart failure may occur. Children with CHD show failure to thrive with stunted physical growth and mental insufficiency, due to lowered blood flow to the organs and low oxygen concentration in the blood. Surgical correction, if done in time, can often reverse these changes to allow for normal, healthy development.

Due to the large variety of congenital defects, only a selected number of diseases will be described here. Treatment will be discussed in this chapter as well as in Chapter 9 ("External and Implantable Cardiac Devices") and Chapter 10 ("Surgical Treatment for Heart Disease").

Patent Foramen Ovale

Blood from the mother containing oxygen and nutrients passes through the umbilical cord to nourish the fetus before birth. Since the fetus is not able to breathe air, there is no point in circulating all the blood through nonfunctioning alveoli in the lungs that are actually clogged with fluid and thus offer a very high resistance to blood flow. There is, therefore, a natural connection between the right and left atria called the *patent foramen ovale* (PFO) that looks like a flap made by two curtains. This opening allows blood entering the right atrium to bypass the lungs and flow from the right heart and into the left heart. A foramen ovale typically closes shortly after birth or within the first few years of life. However, in 25 percent of people the PFO remains open well into adulthood and never closes. A PFO does not ordinarily cause any problems, even if it persists into adulthood, though blood may leak over from the right to the left atrium during coughing or straining due to changes in pressure inside the atria. The actual volume of flow is small and shunting of blood does not lead to cyanotic heart disease, as described above. People with a PFO without complications can have a normal life span and often they live an untroubled life. However, sometimes a PFO can predispose to serious problems, namely strokes, as described below. In fact, a PFO is found in 40 percent of unexplained stroke patients, the majority of whom are below 60 years of age.

When clots form in the veins of the legs or pelvis under certain conditions (venous thrombosis), they may detach and travel to the heart. Normally, such clots travel to the right atrium, the right ventricle, and to the lungs where they are trapped. No great harm results if the clots are small. However, if the clots travel from the right atrium of the heart to the left side through a PFO, they accidentally get into the arterial system. Such clots can obstruct an artery and cause sudden blockage of blood flow. A clot that travels to the brain results in a stroke or a transient ischemic attack (TIA). The person develops sudden numbness or loss of movement in a limb, loss of speech or vision in one eye, or loss of consciousness. If such a clot travels to the coronary arteries, a myocardial infarction occurs. In such cases, a diagnosis is made by an arteriogram and the clot is treated by angioplasty to open the coronary artery. If a limb artery is blocked, there is sudden pain when blood flow is cut off, and the clot has to be removed surgically.

The diagnosis of PFO is made by Doppler echocardiography and a "bubble study" that shows abnormal flow from the right atrium into the left atrium. An agitated saline solution containing air bubbles is injected into a vein, and during straining or coughing, the bubbles can be seen streaming across the PFO from the right to the left atrium. The pathway taken by the bubbles visualized on the echocardiogram confirms the diagnosis. Treatment consists of placing the patient on an anticoagulant such as aspirin, warfarin (Coumadin), or clopidogrel (Plavix) for a lifetime to prevent clotting of blood. If the person is asymptomatic, a PFO found incidentally during echocardiography is generally not treated surgically and anticoagulation need not be performed in most cases due to the hazards of long-term anticoagulation. This decision is a risk-benefit analysis, as treatment with a powerful anticoagulant such as warfarin is associated with serious bleeding complications. It is not known if treatment with aspirin, clopidogrel, and other antiplatelet drugs is beneficial in this situation to prevent embolism, and these drugs are currently not recommended routinely.

If the PFO is large and/or embolization has occurred, the opening can be closed surgically or using a percutaneous catheter technique. These procedures are discussed in more detail in Chapters 9 and 10.

Atrial Septal Defect

One of the most common kinds of CHD is *atrial septal defect* (ASD) occurring in 1 out of 1,500 births. In an ASD, there is a hole in the septum between the left atrium and the right atrium. The atrial and ventricular septa are supposed to grow completely in fetal life, so the heart ultimately becomes divided into four chambers. However, the walls are not always completely constructed by the time the baby is born, and a connection is left between the adjoining chambers. Often, septal development continues after birth and the defect is closed by the age of five or six. In some cases, holes of variable size may be persistent, and if the defect is large, significant shunting of blood occurs. Patients with ASD remain asymptomatic for long periods of time as long as there is no shunt reversal. Once shunt reversal occurs, venous blood is pumped from the right side of the heart to the left side through the hole and by this time it is too late to repair the defect. In many such cases, right-sided heart failure occurs when pulmonary hypertension progresses as the right ventricle can no longer sustain its pumping action against the high pressures in the lung circulation.

Since ASD is generally acyanotic, it is often missed on clinical examination, and it is largely silent on auscultation because the flow of blood between the chambers is very quiet due to low pressures in both atrial chambers. The initial suspicion that the patient has an ASD arises when the patient presents with shortness of breath or congestive heart failure. The diagnosis is made by Doppler echocardiography and cardiac catheterization. Even if the ASD is asymptomatic, it should generally be closed though the person may have no symptoms. If repair is not done, pulmonary hypertension will result over time with symptoms of shortness of breath, and life span may be shortened.

Ventricular Septal Defect

A ventricular septal defect (VSD) occurs when the ventricular septum does not close off completely to separate the two ventricles completely, so that a direct connection exists between the two ventricles. The panel on the left in Figure 7.1 shows the location of the VSD in the mid-portion of the ventricular septum. The

Congenital heart disease
Ventricular septal defect

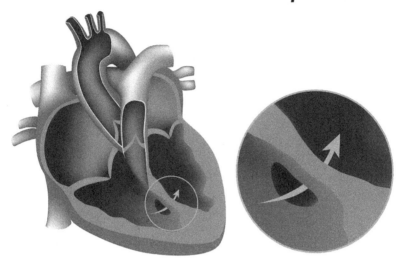

Figure 7.1 Ventricular septal defect (VSD). The panel on the left shows the location of the VSD in the septum between the right and left ventricles. The panel on the right shows the direction of blood flow from the right to the left ventricle. © Alila07/Dreamstime.com.

panel on the right shows the direction of blood flow from the right ventricle to the left ventricle during shunt reversal as described later. The usual pattern of flow in VSD is in the opposite direction.

This form of CHD comprises 30 percent of all cardiac defects, occurring in about 1 out of every 500 births. The ventricular septum is made up of two sections: a membranous upper third and a muscular lower two thirds. If the membranous part does not develop normally, a hole is left between the two ventricles, reminiscent of the heart in a crocodilian reptile. About 80 percent of VSDs are of this type.

Diagnosis is easily made clinically as there is a very characteristic loud, blowing *crescendo-decrescendo murmur* heard during ventricular systole all over the chest. The diagnosis is confirmed by Doppler echocardiography or cardiac catheterization.

Closure of the VSD can be done percutaneously using a device inserted though a catheter, as described for ASD. Surgical closure is the standard method for large VSDs, with the patient on a heart-lung machine, using a Dacron graft or a piece of the patient's own pericardium stitched in place with fine sutures. There is a risk of damage to the electrical conduction system during surgery, and heart block can occur. This complication occurs as the atrioventricular node is close to the upper part of the septum and as the bundle branches are embedded in the septum. If heart block occurs, a permanent pacemaker needs to be implanted following surgery. With very small VSDs that are of pinhole size, there is the option to leave it untreated.

Generally, VSD is acyanotic in the early stages, as the flow of blood is from the left ventricle to the right side of the heart. However, when there is significant shunting of blood from the left to the right side of the heart, the pressure in the pulmonary circulation builds up over time to produce pulmonary hypertension. This condition gradually results in the pressures on the right side of the heart becoming abnormally high and eventually exceeding the pressure in the left ventricle. At this point, there is shunt reversal and blood flows from the right ventricle to the left ventricle, as shown in Figure 7.1. When shunt reversal occurs, the person becomes very symptomatic and it is often too late to close the VSD, and the situation becomes rather grim with poor long-term survival.

Atrioventricular Canal Defect

A rather rare and very complex defect called the atrioventricular (AV) canal defect is seen when an ASD, a VSD, and abnormalities of the mitral and tricuspid valves occur together right in the center of the heart. This condition is seen in 20 percent of patients with Down syndrome, or in 1 out of 5,000 births. The condition allows mixing of blood in all four chambers and needs correction within the first six months of life to close the abnormal connections. A variety of complicated procedures have been devised to treat this complex condition surgically, as it is a serious defect that is not compatible with a long life.

Patent Ductus Arteriosus

Another well-known form of congenital abnormality is *patent ductus arteriosus* (PDA). This is a connection via a channel between the aorta and the pulmonary artery, which lie close together. Normally, this channel shunts blood pumped from the right ventricle away from the lungs in fetal life and into the aorta, and it closes off soon after birth. However, in some babies, it remains open for many years and into adulthood, producing a loud rumbling and continuous sound called a *machinery murmur*, heard all over the chest.

The high pressure in the aorta shunts blood into the pulmonary artery and overloads the lungs, causing oxygenated blood to mix with deoxygenated blood if a PDA persists into adulthood. Over time, the blood pressure in the lungs builds up due to years of high blood flow and pulmonary hypertension results. Gradually, due to the high pressure in the lung circulation, the direction of blood reverses itself so that the blue deoxygenated blood gets into the general circulation and the baby becomes a "blue baby." By then, the child is in serious trouble as its health has deteriorated to the point where closing off the shunt may not be helpful. Therefore, early intervention to close off the shunt is necessary.

Premature infants, rubella, and Down's syndrome are risk factors for PDA. The diagnosis is made by clinical examination and by Doppler echocardiography. This condition always needs to be treated and surgical ligation of the PDA can be done. However, to avoid surgery a steel coil covered with Dacron can also be inserted through a catheter to cause clotting and closure of the PDA. Injection of medications such as indomethacin and prostaglandin E can also be used to close off the PDA medically and without surgical intervention.

Tetralogy of Fallot

The most common cause of cyanotic heart disease at birth is the *Tetralogy of Fallot* (ToF), which is seen in 400 out of 1 million births, causing about 60–70 percent of all so-called blue babies. It is associated with deletions in chromosome 22. In this malformation, the aorta "overrides" both the left and right ventricles (when normally it connects only with the left side) so that mixing of venous and arterial blood occurs. There is also pulmonary valve narrowing and ventricular septal defect in ToF. In some cases, there is an atrial septal defect or other cardiac abnormalities. All of these defects alter pressures within the heart so that there is chamber enlargement due to increased loads of blood volume on the heart. Such enlargement leads to inefficient pumping action of the heart and to congestive heart failure. A complex surgical operation is necessary to fix this condition.

Biscuspid Aortic Valve

The aortic valve has three leaflets, but in 1–2 percent of people, two of the leaflets or cusps fuse into a single leaflet. This produces a valve that is bicuspid. The condition is twice as common in men as in women for unknown reasons, and there may be a familial incidence as the occurrence of the condition increases to 10 percent in relatives of afflicted people. It is thought that the condition is inherited as an autosomal dominant gene with incomplete penetrance. This condition is sometimes associated with aortic coarctation and with expansion (aneurysm) of the root of the aorta.

Generally, there is no major problem with the functioning of the valve, though a harsh ejection murmur is often heard across the valve on auscultation. However, the valve often becomes calcified and narrowed when the person is in the fifth and sixth decades of life. Thus, it is necessary for the person to see a cardiologist and have echocardiograms done on an annual basis. This condition may require valve replacement as discussed in Chapters 4 and 10.

Coarctation of the Aorta

Coarctation, strictly speaking, is not a congenital *heart* disease, as it occurs in the aorta and not in the heart itself. However, it is sometimes associated with mitral and aortic valve disease, VSD, and PDA. Coarctation is also seen more frequently in children born to diabetic mothers and in Turner syndrome.

In this condition, there is an hourglass crimping of the aorta that leads to the obstruction of blood flow. Coarctation may occur anywhere along the length of the aorta. If the obstruction is present after the arteries to the arms branch off, blood pressure in the arms will be elevated, and the pressure in the legs will be normal. Taking blood pressure in the arms and legs and noticing a significant difference between the two readings can make the diagnosis. Sometimes the obstruction occurs in a location on the aorta between the origins of the artery to the right arm and the left arm. In such a case, there is a large difference between the blood pressure readings in the two arms.

If the condition is not treated, the left ventricle enlarges and hypertrophies and may even fail to pump properly. Rarely, there may be aortic dissection where the vessel splits lengthwise due to the elevated pressure. The diagnosis is made through CT scanning, MRI, or angiography. Treatment consists of removing the obstruction surgically and inserting a Gore-Tex graft. Sometimes, angioplasty can be done to dilate the narrowed segment.

Hypoplastic Heart Syndromes

Hypoplasia refers to the underdevelopment of the muscle of the right or left ventricle and is generally a cyanotic heart defect. Though this is a rare condition, it is one of the most serious forms of CHD. It is called *hypoplastic left heart syndrome* when it affects the left side of the heart and *hypoplastic right heart syndrome* when it affects the right. This condition leads to only one side of the heart being able to pump blood to the body and lungs effectively. In both conditions, the presence of a patent ductus arteriosus is vital to the infant's ability to survive until emergency heart surgery can be performed. When hypoplasia affects the right side of the heart, a patent foramen ovale keeps blood flowing from the right heart to the left heart allowing forward flow through the left ventricle in the short term. Without these pathways blood cannot circulate to the body or the lungs, depending on which side of the heart is affected.

The treatment consists of complex surgical procedures done very early in life to redirect blood flow in the heart. Alternatively, cardiac transplantation is done to replace the entire heart.

Transposition of the Great Arteries

Transposition of the great arteries (TGA) is a form of cyanotic heart disease that occurs when the large arteries of the heart are connected to the wrong chambers. Normally, the aorta comes off the left ventricle and the pulmonary artery comes off the right ventricle. However, in TGA, the positions are switched. This condition is often associated with patent foramen ovale, atrial and ventricular septal defects, and patent ductus arteriosus. This condition is not compatible with life long-term, as the venous blood is not oxygenated since it leaves the right ventricle through the aorta to return to the body without ever going through the lungs. However, life is sustained for a short period as blood crosses over from one side of the heart to the other through a patent foramen ovale or some other defect, and partial oxygenation is achieved.

This condition is seen with greater frequency with maternal diabetes and in certain genetic abnormalities. The diagnosis is made by echocardiography, MRI, or CT scanning. Surgery is necessary to switch the arteries to their correct anatomical positions or the child will eventually die.

SIGNS AND SYMPTOMS

Despite children being examined at birth, many grow into adulthood before congenital heart defects are discovered during a routine examination. In early childhood, a child may develop symptoms such as palpitations, fainting, breathlessness, and he may have blue lips and fingertips if there is right-to-left shunting of blood. Because the organs do not receive 100 percent oxygenation, the brain and other organs to not develop normally because of lack of enough oxygen. The child is physically stunted in growth and becomes short of breath easily, especially during exertion. Children with serious CHD often assume a squatting position as it takes less effort than standing up, and their lips and fingertips turn blue if they are light-skinned. There is also often delayed mental development because of inadequate oxygenation to the brain. Development is improved when surgical correction is undertaken.

In some cases, usually in adults, a heart defect is discovered when a presumably healthy person suddenly develops a stroke, as described earlier. When an echocardiogram is done, a previously unsuspected atrial septal defect or a patent foramen ovale is discovered.

DIAGNOSIS AND TREATMENT

Clinical Examination

An initial history and clinical examination is essential to identify the cause of symptoms. Often, the parent notices shortness of breath, fainting spells, cyanosis, failure to thrive, or failure to achieve normal developmental milestones. Auscultation of the heart will provide clues to certain conditions, as there are classical auscultatory findings in conditions such as ventricular septal defect and patent ductus arteriosus. Some murmurs are so distinctive that they are virtually diagnostic.

In the newborn, babies are examined at birth and an *Apgar score* is evaluated. This score, devised by Dr. Virginia Apgar (1909-1974), consists of evaluating five signs within five minutes of birth: pulse rate, breathing, skin color, response to stimulation, and muscle tone. A score of zero (no pulse or breathing, blue skin color, no response to stimulation, and no muscle tone) means the baby is dead or practically dead and may need revival. A score of 7–10 is considered to be in the normal range. A physical examination done in babies with a low Apgar score will often show cardiac developmental abnormalities.

Diagnostic Testing

Normal human gestation is nine months, and if babies are born prematurely, their organs may not be fully developed. Prenatal diagnosis is also now possible since echocardiograms through the mother's abdomen can be done as early as at 14 weeks of fetal life. A diagnosis of severe cardiac malformation can therefore be made *in utero*. In such cases, immediate postdelivery care can be given in the newborn intensive care unit with special monitoring and supplemental oxygen. Early surgery can also be planned in cases where the baby would die if this were not done.

Diagnostic testing in both children and adults consists of echocardiography, magnetic resonance imaging (MRI), computer tomography (CT) scanning, cardiac catheterization, and angiography to identify abnormalities in the heart and the great vessels. These studies are generally definitive and will confirm the clinical diagnosis by identifying the abnormal structures.

Genetic Testing

Genetic testing is done using blood, skin, and buccal mucosa from the inside of the cheeks. Such testing can be done for screening for genetically transmitted diseases in children and adults if a genetically transmitted disease is suspected or to screen for carriers of a defective gene.

Prenatal testing is used to detect changes in genes or chromosomes in a fetus before birth. This type of testing is offered to couples with a high risk of having a baby with a genetic defect. Testing cannot possibly identify all possible inherited disorders, but can help a couple if they wish to abort the pregnancy. Genetic testing can be done by amniocentesis during pregnancy. A local anesthetic is given to the mother in order to reduce the pain felt during the insertion of the needle used to withdraw amniotic fluid. A needle is inserted through the mother's abdominal wall, through the wall of the uterus, to penetrate the amniotic sac containing fluid using ultrasound guidance. About 20 milliliters of amniotic fluid is extracted and the fetal cells are isolated from the sample. The cells are grown in a culture medium, then chemically fixed and stained for analysis under a microscope. The stained chromosomes can be seen and are examined for chromosomal abnormalities. A diagnosis for Down syndrome or Turner syndrome or other genetic abnormalities can thus be made prenatally. The doctor can then counsel the parents as to the best course of action. Today, many large children's hospitals have geneticists on staff who provide prenatal and postnatal counseling.

ETHICAL AND MORAL ISSUES

The ability to detect diseases with the aid of advanced technology is a great boon enjoyed by many people in the modern era. Genetic counseling is now routinely performed in many major medical centers to screen for genetically transmitted diseases when such diseases are suspected. However, after the diagnosis of heart defects or a serious genetic abnormality is made in the unborn baby, the parents often face a conundrum. In some cases, the fetus simply cannot survive to maturity and many die soon after birth.

However, difficult ethical and moral issues arise if the diagnosis of a serious cardiac or genetic defect is made in a fetus before birth. Since abortion is now legal in many countries, the parents have a choice whether to keep the baby or to abort it. The difficulty lies in predicting with any degree of accuracy if the baby will thrive, the amount of care it will need, and the expense of such an endeavor. The threshold for decision making is very difficult in many cases, especially in genetic abnormalities such as Down or Turner syndrome where, in most cases, the baby will survive, but will have subnormal intelligence. The question is whether an abortion should be done. While the law is clear in the United States and in many Western countries that the woman has the right to choose for herself, the deeper moral question is whether fetuses with potentially subnormal intelligence have a right to life.

Another difficult decision is whether carriers of genes that cause serious inherited disorders should reproduce and become parents. If the decision is made to have children, the child may have to be aborted if it is abnormal, or the child will become a carrier for the defective gene. These decisions are extremely personal and often cause intense psychological distress for the parents, and especially for the mother. The decision is more complicated when there is a multiple pregnancy where one fetus is abnormal and selective abortion may have to be performed. Mothers report feelings of guilt when they have to sacrifice the fetus that is defective. In many centers today, genetic counseling is coupled with psychological counseling to help parents cope with these difficult problems.

Another new ethical challenge arises when the parents of an affected child deliberately conceive a second child for the specific reason to obtain stem cells or genetic material to be used to treat a previously conceived child afflicted by a genetic disease. Stem cell therapy raises other moral and ethical issues. Stem cells are primordial cells that can become any specialized tissue in the body and replace or regenerate parts of a particular organ. Such cells may be derived from adult stem cells or from fetuses. Currently, the use of fetal stem cells is debated because it means that the fetus has to be sacrificed. Opponents of abortion feel very strongly that it is morally wrong to abort a fetus specifically to obtain stem cells. The issue of genetic manipulation to treat such cardiac conditions is dealt with in Chapter 13.

SUMMARY

Congenital heart disease often occurs as a result of genetic problems or environmental risk factors experienced by the mother during pregnancy. Chromosomal and genetic abnormalities occur as a consequence of exposure to certain viruses, radiation, and chemicals. These factors can give rise to assorted genetic malformations of the heart. In some types of CHD, the diagnosis is not immediately obvious at the time of birth or in early childhood, as symptoms manifest only later in life. In some types of CHD, single lesions occur, but in some cases, complex types of abnormalities coexist. Some of these defects are not compatible with life, while others will shorten life unless corrective action is taken. Most heart defects are associated with genetic abnormalities, and new links are being discovered with genomic analysis. New treatments are also being devised for complex heart defects and early intervention is helping people survive longer.

8

Tests for Heart Disease

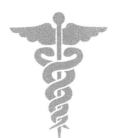

Cardiology is the most technologically intensive discipline in medicine. Today almost every function of the heart can be measured with special tests, many of which will be described in this chapter. The heart is a two-stage pump that is both a mechanical and an electrical organ with its own inbuilt electrical circuitry. This electromechanical organ is much like an internal combustion engine. In such engines there is an electrical spark that ignites gasoline within a chamber that converts energy into mechanical action. When functioning normally, the heart's electrical system makes it pump at a regular rate. When cardiac disorders occur, there may be problems that affect the electrical components of the heart, or there may be problems with the mechanical parts of the heart.

In diseases that affect the electrical system of the heart, the pulse rate changes and in many cases, the person feels a thumping in the heart, and erratic racing, or slowing of the heartbeat. When the heart rate accelerates rapidly or when the pulse slows down greatly, the person develops dizziness or fainting due to lack of blood flow to the brain. In some cases the heart goes into cardiac arrest and the person needs to be resuscitated. The commonest cause of death in humans is an electrical disruption of the heart and not mechanical failure.

When the mechanical pumping action of the heart is significantly impaired, the person feels short of breath, or a sense of great fatigue sets in. In fact, fatigue is one of the most common symptoms of coronary disease and congenital heart disease. Weakness and fainting occurs because there is decreased blood flow from the heart, so not enough oxygen is carried to the body, resulting in a lack of oxygenation of the muscles that carry out normal physical activity. Fatigue is a very common symptom in heart disease, but since this is a ubiquitous symptom it is not very specific to heart disease.

Doctors make a preliminary clinical diagnosis based on the combination of symptoms reported by the patient and a physical examination. They then decide which of several tests need to be done to make a more precise diagnosis. These tests can be divided into three groups:

- Tests that examine the electrical functioning of the heart (i.e., the rhythm of the heart)
- Tests that examine the anatomical and mechanical functioning of the heart (i.e., blood flow to the heart and the pumping action of the heart)
- Radiological studies of the heart

In some tests (e.g., *cardiac catheterization*), there is an overlap between these three types of tests. Very often, cardiologists also divide tests into two categories: *noninvasive tests* (electrocardiogram [EKG], stress tests, echocardiography, magnetic resonance imaging) and *invasive tests* (cardiac catheterization and cardiac electrophysiology). Most often, when there is no great urgency, noninvasive tests are done first to make a diagnosis as they are easier to do in a doctor's office or as an outpatient and as they are less costly and cause few complications. If noninvasive tests do not provide an answer, invasive tests will have to be done directly on the heart and its blood vessels. Such tests require hospitalization and are not only costly, as they require more sophisticated equipment, but they can also occasionally cause serious complications. When making a diagnosis of heart disease, no one test is a stand-alone test. In most cases, a series of tests is done to arrive at a diagnosis and to fashion a treatment plan.

TESTS THAT EXAMINE ELECTRICAL FUNCTIONS OF THE HEART

Electrocardiography

The electrocardiogram (EKG or ECG) has become the most widely used tool in making an initial diagnosis of heart disease since it was introduced into clinical use by Willem Einthoven in 1903. No matter what the disease is thought to be, it provides useful general information on the electrical activity of the heart and can, at the same time, provide indirect information on mechanical function. The EKG takes just about a minute to record, and it is, therefore, a kind of snapshot of the heart in a moment in time.

The entire EKG is made of 12 different parts (also called "leads") that give an *electrical view* of the heart by looking at it from 12 different angles. This virtual electrical view of the heart is commonly referred to as a *12-lead EKG*, and it is constructed by attaching electrodes to different parts of the body. Each lead functions like an electrical coordinate that corresponds to a specific anatomical region of the heart. By observing which particular leads are affected in a 12-lead EKG, a doctor can estimate roughly where in the heart a particular problem may be located.

As discussed in Chapter 1, Einthoven named the electrical waves P, Q, R, S, and T waves. Since the waves represent various kinds of electrical activity occurring in different parts of the heart, abnormalities in the shape and configuration of the P-wave, the QRS-complex, the ST-segment, the QT-interval, and the T-wave, it is possible to make a preliminary diagnosis. The effects of drugs, electrolytes, and hypothermia on the heart can also be deduced from the EKG and corrective action taken. In the case of a myocardial infarction, a diagnosis can be made as to which area of the heart is, or was, affected by a disease process. Acutely occurring damage and old areas of damage each present a distinctive pattern on the EKG. It is possible also to estimate roughly how much heart muscle is affected or damaged during a myocardial infarction. During the evolution of a myocardial infarction, the progress of the attack can be charted by doing serial EKGs at regular intervals. A doctor can tell if a particular area is becoming damaged, or if a myocardial infarction is enlarging, even as it is occurring. If the area was already damaged years ago and has healed, the abnormality shows up with a different pattern and is recognized as a scar from an old myocardial infarction that does not require active treatment.

During anginal attacks, when there is no damage to heart muscle, the pattern is different from myocardial infarction. This helps differentiate the pain from angina from that of infarction. The doctor already knows what a "normal" EKG looks like in most people, so these changes strongly suggest that a heart attack is occurring in the inferior (bottom) part of the heart. Even after a hundred years, the EKG is therefore the single most important test to do to diagnose a myocardial infarction, commonly known as a "heart attack."

The EKG can also be helpful in diagnosing heart rhythm abnormalities. If a person has palpitations and the rhythm abnormality lasts for a long time or is frequent enough, a single EKG can make the diagnosis immediately. This test is very useful as an initial screening device, but if the abnormal rhythm occurs infrequently, an EKG will be unlikely to show it as it charts the rhythm for less than a minute and other tests are needed. In such cases, EKG monitoring over an extended period is necessary.

Specialized forms of the EKG analysis are built into many EKG machines today. These computer programs include analysis of the T-wave to measure a phenomenon called *T-wave alternans,* where there are beat-to-beat alterations in the height or shape of the T-wave on the EKG. This kind of variation is seen in patients who may be vulnerable to cardiac arrest. Another specialized EKG is the signal-averaged electrocardiogram (SAECG). The SAECG is done like a regular EKG but over 7–10 minutes and then overlapped multiple times using a special computer program. After filtering out extraneous interference so that small variations at the end of the QRS complex are removed, the QRS is printed on a larger than normal scale to show "late potentials" in the terminal part of the QRS complex. This process may reveal susceptibility to cardiac arrest from ventricular fibrillation. Though easily available, it has not seen widespread application, as most electrophysiologists prefer direct cardiac testing to make a diagnosis.

Holter Monitoring

Heart rhythm abnormalities are often not present all the time, so it is difficult to know what the problem is when a person complains of infrequent palpitations. The regular EKG contains only about 60 seconds of information, and this is too short period of time to pick up abnormal heart beats that occur intermittently. In order to find out how the heart is beating when the person goes about normal activities, such as walking, eating, sleeping, or exercising, more extended recording of heart rhythm is needed. This kind of monitoring is called Holter monitoring, named for Norman Holter (1914–1983), the biophysicist who devised the original equipment for this test.

This test is done with a tape or digital recorder that continuously records and stores the heart rhythm. Adhesive electrodes are attached to the chest and connected to the recording device that is worn on a belt or holster for 24–48 hours. The information is downloaded and played back on a computer that displays heart rate and rhythm, and any abnormal heartbeats. The data are analyzed on a computer that is programmed with automated algorithms that allows it to chart trends in heart rate and to quantify the different types of abnormal beats. The automated program determines whether the heart is beating normally or abnormally and how often abnormal events occur. A human reader has to oversee this process as it is not a perfect system and errors can occur even with the best computer programs.

It is actually very common to find extra beats (*atrial* or *ventricular premature beats*) in a normal person. It is just as common to find short bursts of abnormal beats even in normal hearts, and most of these do not require treatment. In people with heart disease, the doctor has to make a decision whether these beats are dangerous to health or whether they should be observed carefully over time. This is a clinical decision that depends on many factors, including the general health of the person and the physical condition of the heart as determined by other tests.

Telemetry of the EKG

Telemetry is a wireless method of transmitting heartbeats to a central nursing station by a transmitter attached by adhesive electrodes to the chest by electrical leads. This method allows observation of the heart rhythm following a myocardial infarction or following high-risk surgery when there may be rhythm disorders.

Sometimes a person reports an erratic pulse, but a normal EKG or Holter monitoring does not show what is wrong. In other cases, a patient may have fainting spells and a heart rhythm disorder is suspected. In these cases, it is not immediately clear what has happened, nor is it obvious that the heart is the culprit. To uncover the problem, the patient is hospitalized and EKG monitoring done by telemetry. Such observation alone may provide useful information if the patient has another fainting spell and this can be correlated with a heart rhythm abnormality. In such cases, invasive testing as described below is needed. If the fainting spell or dizziness while under continuous observation cannot be correlated with a rhythm abnormality, a neurological or other cause must be sought.

Electrophysiological Testing

In many cases, an EKG, in whatever form as described above, is insufficient to provide the necessary information. This is the case when the abnormal rhythm is episodic and does not occur spontaneously in order to be captured by a regular EKG. In order to provoke the abnormal heart rhythm that is suspected to occur episodically, the heart undergoes provocative electrical testing called an *electrophysiological study* (*EPS*). This test is done very much the same way as a cardiac catheterization, in a special sterile laboratory equipped with radiographic equipment, resuscitation equipment, an electrical stimulator, monitoring devices, and recording and display devices.

A catheter that has two or more platinum electrodes at the tip is threaded into the heart through a vein. Actually, several such catheters may be placed in several different locations in the heart to record electrical potentials, in different locations such as the right atrium, the right ventricle, the coronary sinus, or the Bundle of His. The intracardiac EKG recorded from these catheters within the heart is displayed on multiple large screens.

These catheters, placed inside the heart, record electrical activity not seen in the surface EKG. They provide more accurate information on how electrical impulses are generated and conducted inside the heart. The activation sequences are used to produce an electrical map of the heart. Such *electrical mapping* provides precise measurements to evaluate conduction times within the heart and help localize abnormalities within the atria, the ventricles, and the conduction system of the heart. The heart can be artificially paced at high rates to elicit the specific electrical abnormality, instead of waiting for it to occur spontaneously. If there is, for example, electrical blockage in cardiac impulse conduction within the heart, provocative testing can bring the problem to the surface so that a diagnosis can be made. This kind of impaired conduction may not be present all the time, which is why a regular EKG cannot always provide an accurate diagnosis.

Besides measuring the EKG from inside the heart, small electrical impulses can also be discharged into the heart via these catheters directly onto the inside surface of the heart. Using an automatic computer program to deliver the impulse, the intensity and location of the impulse during the cardiac cycle can be varied in a sequential manner. Such programmed electrical stimulation can provoke spurts of ventricular tachycardia (VT) or even ventricular fibrillation (VF). The ultimate objective is to discover if the heart is electrically unstable and vulnerable to cardiac arrest. If the heart cannot be easily provoked into a life-threatening rhythm, then no treatment is needed. If, however, there is electrical instability by electrophysiological testing, drug treatment may be given, or implantation of a defibrillator performed.

Since EPS is an invasive test, it is possible for serious side effects such as bleeding, infection, and rarely, ventricular fibrillation and death, to occur. Though the risk of complications from EPS is low, it is reserved for arrhythmias that are difficult to diagnose or rhythms that are potentially life-threatening. This procedure is also used for the treatment of difficult arrhythmias using electrical ablation of conduction system pathways to cure certain arrhythmias, as described later.

TESTS THAT EXAMINE ANATOMICAL AND MECHANICAL FUNCTIONS OF THE HEART

Exercise Stress Testing

Exercise stress testing (commonly called a *stress test*) is done to check the mechanical functioning of the heart and the physical endurance of a person.

The length of time a person can exercise is not only a measure of the muscular strength of a person, but also a measure of heart function. The duration of exercise is an excellent low-cost method to predict the state of the heart using only a treadmill (or a stationary bicycle) and an EKG machine. Exercise stress may also occasionally expose the presence of exercise-induced arrhythmias.

Rationale

Following certain standardized criteria, the test is used primarily to discover if the person has coronary artery disease. A stress test is done when a person has symptoms of chest pain or discomfort, fatigue or shortness of breath and CAD is suspected. The exercise test by itself cannot make a definitive diagnosis of coronary artery disease. The series of EKGs done during the test may show changes during the test that *suggest* that the person *probably* has CAD. The accuracy of the test depends on the pre-test probability of CAD. If the person has a good history for angina, is in an older age group, and has risk factors for CAD, the test is accurate about 80 percent of the time in predicting the diagnosis as CAD. If the person is young and has atypical chest pain, a negative test has a high probability of predicting that he does not have CAD.

Stress tests are often done before embarking on a strenuous exercise program, in people in high physical stress occupations, and before major operations, if the patient is in an older age group. The test is also done to discover if a patient with high-risk arrhythmias can exercise safely.

The principle of the test is that as exercise level is increased, the heart muscle consumes more and more oxygen. If there are serious blockages in the arteries feeding blood to the heart, this leads to an insufficient oxygen supply to the heart. The result is that the oxygen requirement outstrips the supply available, leading to a condition called *cardiac ischemia*. This condition can cause chest pain as the level of effort during the stress test is increased, and requires the test to be stopped.

Method and Equipment

The objective of a cardiac stress test is to determine how much effort a person can expend before stopping due to fatigue or due to the onset of cardiovascular symptoms. This test examines the response of heart rate (HR), blood pressure (BP), and the EKG to exercise stress. In the United States, most exercise laboratories use a protocol based on a motorized treadmill, while in Europe and many other countries, a stationary bicycle is more commonly used. During the treadmill test, the person walks on a moving belt, and the speed and elevation are automatically increased gradually at three-minute increments. The bicycle protocol is similar, and the person rides a stationary bicycle ergometer with progressively increasing resistance applied to the wheel to increase the effort expended. Such tests are very safe when conducted under medical supervision with oxygen, drugs, and resuscitation equipment available in case an emergency occurs. The personnel present are trained in basic and advanced life support. A defibrillator is on hand in case of a cardiac arrest, though this event occurs only very rarely with exercise testing.

Before the test is done, electrodes are attached to the chest to track the EKG continuously on a monitor during and following exercise. A resting EKG tracing is obtained before starting exercise, and an EKG is then done every three minutes. The blood pressure is measured at rest and every three minutes also at the same time as the EKG. The last EKG is done at peak exercise. The test is done to the point of exhaustion, or it is halted when the person says he wishes to stop because of fatigue, chest discomfort, or pain. This type of stress test is called a *maximal stress test*. Sometimes the doctor will observe changes in the EKG or a decrease in blood pressure and stop the test. The EKG done at peak exercise is compared to the EKG obtained at rest to compare them for changes that suggest ischemia. During the recovery period that lasts 10 minutes following exercise, an EKG is done every 3 minutes to track any late changes that occur post-exercise. Changes in the EKG during exercise are compared to the resting EKG, and this will help make the diagnosis of coronary artery disease if there are important changes observed in the ST-segment during exercise.

The duration of exercise, and the heart rate and blood pressure responses to exercise, will vary by age and sex. To get an idea what "normal" stress test results look like, exercise stress tests were done on thousands of healthy people to determine responses to exercise of heart rate, blood pressure, and EKG in men and women in different age groups. The data on heart rate and blood pressure on these healthy volunteers were summarized in tables and *normograms* (graphs) generated to delineate patients by age, sex, and duration of exercise. In this way, a patient's test results can be compared to a person of similar age and sex to determine how much the test subject deviates from the norm, in order to help make a more accurate diagnosis.

Quite often in heart disease, there is the early onset of fatigue or shortness of breath (dyspnea), rather than the onset of chest pain during exercise. Fatigue and shortness of breath are called *anginal equivalents* as they are proxies for angina in CAD. Fatigue and dyspnea on exertion often come on before there is angina. However, both fatigue and dyspnea are very common nonspecific symptoms that are often due to lack of exercise conditioning and common to other conditions as well. Fatigue alone in someone who is out of shape is not a reliable indicator of heart disease. There have to be concomitant EKG changes to make a more definitive diagnosis of ischemia. Another sign heart disease could be present occurs when there are inadequate increases in heart rate and blood pressure during exercise. This feature is called an *abnormal hemodynamic response*, and it tells the doctor that something is wrong with the functioning of the heart and the circulation.

Interpretation

Interpretation of a cardiac stress test is based on symptoms, EKG changes and the hemodynamic response to stress. When the test is completed, the doctor compares the heart rate and blood pressure at peak exercise with a comparable group of healthy people of the same sex and age obtained from the normogram chart. In patients with heart disease, the duration of exercise and the heart rate and blood pressure at the maximum level of exercise are all lower than in normal people. The EKG measured at peak exercise is compared to the EKG taken at baseline before exercise was started. In many cases of heart disease, the EKG also becomes progressively abnormal as exercise proceeds.

The language used by cardiologists to describe the results of a stress test may appear a little odd to the layperson. When the test is normal, it is called a *negative test* and what it means is that the test is negative for ischemia on the EKG. Of course, this is a *positive outcome* for the patient. When the test is abnormal, it is called a *positive test*, and this means that the test was *positive for ischemic changes* on the EKG.

There are standard criteria for EKG changes that determine how the diagnosis of cardiac ischemia is made. The principal criterion for ischemia is related to the displacement of the ST-segment of the EKG at the peak of exercise. The normal ST-segment is horizontal and is flat or *isoelectric* when it is normal, as shown in Figure 2.4. During ischemia, the ST-segment may commonly become depressed (or more uncommonly become elevated) and diagnosis depends on the configuration of the ST-segment and the magnitude of the change. The criteria vary depending on whether the ST-segment is horizontal, downsloping, or upsloping. The standard criterion is 1 millimeter or more of horizontal or downsloping depression of the ST-segment for a duration of 80 milliseconds or greater. If the ST-segment is upsloping, the ST-segment should be depressed 1.5–2.0 mm for 80 milliseconds or more to call it a test that is positive for ischemia. Sometimes, ST-segment elevation of 1 millimeter or more for 80 milliseconds or greater is seen when there is ischemia. These EKG changes are more diagnostic of CAD and ischemia if the patient simultaneously reports anginal symptoms, becomes severely short of breath, or has a significant decline in blood pressure at the height of exercise.

In some patients, especially those with diabetes, diagnostic ST-segment changes are seen without chest pain or shortness of breath. This type of response is still considered a positive stress test. The patient is considered to have *silent ischemia* that deserves further investigation.

An exercise stress test does not actually identify the specific artery that is blocked, but in some cases, it gives a rough indication how severe the blockage may be. However, in some patients with advanced and severe CAD, the duration of exercise is severely restricted to 3 minutes or less, sometimes with almost immediate chest pain, and a significant decline in blood pressure along with major changes in many of the EKG leads. In such patients, the conclusion is that there must be severe blockages in one or more major coronary arteries. Such a dramatically positive test demonstrates that the left ventricle is so poorly supplied with blood and oxygen that it fails to mount a satisfactory response to exercise stress so that the patient simply cannot go on exercising.

It should be pointed out that sometimes there are *false positive* stress tests, meaning that the person does not have coronary artery disease, but there are abnormal changes on the EKG as if there were ischemia. Up to 40 percent of all patients tested may have false positive stress tests. Women are more likely than men to have false positive stress tests, and therefore the results have to be interpreted with caution. If the baseline EKG is abnormal to begin with, it is likely that the exercise EKGs will be abnormal and show a false positive result that will lead to an incorrect diagnosis.

A false positive stress test can also occur in patients taking digitalis drugs or certain psychotropic drugs, with a low potassium blood level, and if there is left ventricular hypertrophy or conduction abnormalities in the ventricles. In such cases, the abnormal test is not helpful in making a diagnosis, as the patient may or may not have heart disease. It is more useful to perform a stress test with nuclear imaging, and the results correlated with clinical symptoms in such patients.

A *false negative* test is seen when the person stops exercise prematurely, so that the stress effort is inadequate and the test is deemed *submaximal*. A submaximal test results when a patient gets tired because he is not physically fit, or when he develops leg pain due to peripheral arterial disease, foot or back problems, or arthritis. There are no cardiac symptoms, and the EKGs seem to be perfectly normal with a submaximal test simply because the patient did not exert himself hard enough. The test is reported by the cardiologist as being "a submaximal test that is nondiagnostic due to failure to exercise adequately, and coronary artery disease cannot be ruled out."

In rare instances, serious ventricular arrhythmias and cardiac arrest occur at the height of exercise and the patient collapses so that resuscitation is required. In such cases, the test is positive regardless of what the EKG shows or does not show in terms of the ST-segment changes. It should be emphasized that such a complication is very rare and occurs only once in tens of thousands of tests.

Stress Tests with Imaging

A more advanced form of stress testing is done by taking X-ray images of the heart to make the heart "visible" in order to obtain an assessment of the flow of blood in the heart muscle. This process is done using radiographic techniques to visualize the heart with a special camera that can measure radioactive counts. Testing is done with radioisotopes that are used to "tag" red blood cells that make the heart "light up." These radioactive isotopes (such as thallium, MIBI, or technetium) are injected into the bloodstream so that they attach to red blood cells. The principle is that if blood flow is decreased or absent in a specific region of heart muscle, there will be few or no red blood cells in that particular area of the heart and the heart does not "glow" in that region. Therefore, the radioisotope distributes itself in proportion to the blood flow to the heart. Imaging is done in a resting state (*rest images*) and following the stress test (*stress images*). Therefore, radiographic images of the heart will show a decreased density in damaged areas when the heart is scanned with a special camera.

The actual procedure is to inject the radioisotope so that it circulates and distributes throughout the body. Then, after about 30 minutes, pictures are taken of the heart using a special gamma digital camera. This provides baseline pictures of the heart in several projections. The patient is then "stressed" via exercise. When the person lies down after the termination of exercise, another series of images is made of the heart. The two sets of images, one at baseline and the other post-exercise, are then compared. As the heart may have decreased blood flow to some areas of the ventricular muscle, and increased flow in other areas due to exercise, there is a difference in the amount of blood in each of these areas. This difference is indicated by the density of the radioactive material carried by the blood perfusing the two areas, and this difference in the "glow" can be seen on an X-ray picture of the entire heart. In this manner, one can deduce that a particular area is, or is not, being adequately supplied with blood.

Since we know the anatomy of the coronary arteries, we can deduce that a particular artery to a specific region is blocked, though the artery itself and the degree of blockage cannot actually be seen. If there is a difference between the resting image and the stress image, we know that there is a problem with blood flow to the affected area.

In some cases, a person cannot do physical exercise due to knee or leg problems, such as an amputated leg or leg injuries. In such cases, a medication called dipyrimadole (Persantine) is injected into a vein. The chemical causes *pharmaco-logical stress* by altering blood flow in the coronary arteries. Persantine increases flow in normal coronary arteries and reduces flow distal to partially blocked arter-ies. This effect causes a worsening in the difference in blood flow to the affected ischemic area and to normal heart muscle so that it emulates physical stress. The "rest" and "stress" images are mimicked by taking images of the heart before and after administering the medication.

In some cases, there is a perfusion defect seen in both rest and stress images. When this is discovered, it is assumed that there is scar tissue from a heart attack and the muscle has no blood flow at all, as the muscle is dead. This results in a blank space in the area of dead muscle in the X-ray image of the heart. Therefore, no particular intervention is necessary if the patient is free of symptoms.

Sometimes exercise will result in another kind of problem, which will help to make a diagnosis. While the person is walking or running on the treadmill or cycling on a stationary bicycle, the heart rate speeds up and extra heartbeats may occur. Atrial or ventricular premature beats are very common during exercise. However, when the frequency of such beats increases or become sustained, an ar-rhythmia such as atrial fibrillation, atrial tachycardia, or ventricular tachycardia may occur. Such an exercise-induced arrhythmia may be diagnosed during stress testing and suitable treatment needs to be prescribed.

Complications

Though stress tests are very safe, rarely, complications occur. In severe coronary heart disease, the blood pressure may decline very quickly during exercise, and the patient could come close to fainting if the heart cannot pump enough blood. Even more rarely, a cardiac arrest or myocardial infarction occurs, but it must be emphasized that these events are very rare. It is likely that in such patients, they were probably on the brink of a myocardial infarction and the additional stress provoked the myocardial infarction. In any case, it is much safer to do a stress test under medical supervision, rather than to allow unsupervised strenuous exercise at home or in a gym where the myocardial infarction may have occurred anyway. If such an event occurs, resuscitation equipment is available in the laboratory to im-mediately revive the person and for proper treatment to be provided. Heart attacks occurring during exercise stress testing are rare because the doctor is monitoring the EKG and can stop the test if there are changes that seem to indicate a serious problem. Therefore, patients should be reassured that they are much safer doing EKG monitored exercise in a laboratory under supervision, rather than shoveling snow in cold weather when they could have a myocardial infarction or drop dead.

Cardiac rupture and death has been reported rarely. In such cases, it is likely that the patient was actively undergoing ischemia or early infarction that was not detected, and should possibly not have been subjected to stress testing in the first place.

Echocardiography

Ultrasound, or high-frequency sound that is inaudible to the human ear, is well known in nature as bats and dolphins both use it for navigation. The U.S. Navy started using ultrasound for underwater navigation during the early days of submarine warfare in World War II. The sound used for navigation and detection is called "sonar" (sound navigation and ranging) and it is either *infrasonic* or *ultrasonic*. The human ear can hear from 20 to 20,000 Hertz, and any sound below or above these limits is infrasonic or ultrasonic. The sound used for medical purposes is ultrasonic and is in the range of 2 to 18 megahertz.

Diagnostic ultrasound used for medical purposes is known as *ultrasonography*, and it is used for imaging internal bodily structures. Specialized areas of medicine such as cardiology, obstetrics, gynecology, ophthalmology, and urology rely on this method for clinical diagnostic use. In cardiology, the method is referred to as *echocardiography* and is often simply abbreviated to *echo*. Ultrasonographers or doctors trained in this method perform the test at the bedside or in an outpatient setting.

The test is done using high-frequency sound generated by short electrical pulses that make a piezoelectric transducer ring at a certain frequency. The transducer is encased in a probe and the face of the probe delivers an arc-shaped beam. The ultrasound beam is focused and aimed at an organ, and the reflected sound is converted into an electrical signal by the transducer. This signal is processed to produce a digital image. Sound waves that are reflected from different layers of tissue that have different densities, so that outlines can be defined. For example, heart muscle has a different density when compared to surrounding lung tissue, blood inside the heart, or fluid that accumulates outside the heart during pericardial effusion. This method allows an image to be created of the heart, the great vessels, and any abnormal structures, such as tumors. The image can be stored on videotape, CD, or DVD and played back for analysis.

Measurements are made so that chamber sizes can be determined. Since the normal cardiac chamber sizes are known, comparisons can be made to decide if the heart is enlarged or if the shape of the heart is distorted in some way due to a disease state. If a heart attack (myocardial infarction) has occurred, the area of healed scar tissue does not contract.

Impaired movement of heart muscle can help make a diagnosis of a scar from an old heart attack. The echocardiogram can also be used to study the heart during exercise stress testing. A baseline echocardiogram is done before exercise commences, and this study outlines the shape of the left ventricle at rest. At peak exercise, when the patient has stopped exercising, echocardiographic imaging is done immediately afterward. Ischemic muscle in the left ventricle buckles and moves abnormally when it does not receive adequate blood during exercise as this is a period of high oxygen demand. This study often shows such abnormal movement of heart muscle if there is cardiac ischemia when compared to the baseline study. When the heart rate slows down after exercise stops, the movement of the left ventricle becomes normal again.

Valvular heart disease is best diagnosed by echocardiography as all the cardiac valves can be seen with this study. The study can evaluate the cardiac valves for thickening of the leaflets, for stenosis, regurgitation, rupture, and for vegetations growing on the leaflets. The extent of aortic stenosis can also be calculated using a formula to measure flow across the valve by using Doppler ultrasound to measure the jet stream caused by the ejection of blood across the valve.

Echocardiography is very useful for the diagnosis of pericardial effusion when there is a collection of fluid around the heart. This study is extremely valuable and can be done rapidly in the emergency department to diagnose pericardial effusion that can sometimes be life-threatening. Thickening and calcification of the pericardium in constrictive pericarditis can also be diagnosed by echocardiography.

Cardiac tumors such as left atrial myxoma are very easily diagnosed by echocardiography. Occasionally, the tumor produces a translucent image with an ultrasound study and may be missed at first sight. Clots in the atria and ventricles can also be seen with echocardiography. Such clots are often formed inside the atria during atrial fibrillation, and in the left ventricle after a myocardial infarction.

Echocardiography is often supplemented by a *Doppler flow* study in which the direction and velocity of blood flow is mapped. This study uses sound waves in a different way by drawing on the Doppler effect, where the wavelength of a sound changes when there is movement of the source of the sound. Since blood is in motion in the heart and blood vessels, a sound wave directed at a column of blood can be used to study blood flow. Both pulsed wave and continuous wave Doppler systems are used to convert the sound waves to visual signals that are displayed on a monitor screen. A Doppler flow study shows up in different colors (red or blue) on the screen depending on the direction of blood flow when blood leaks across a valve, or crosses from one chamber to another when there are congenital defects in the heart. The diagnosis of valvular stenosis and regurgitation, patent foramen ovale, atrial, ventricular septal defects, and other defects can be made with this technique.

Cardiac Catheterization

Cardiac catheterization with coronary angiography is an invasive procedure that is the gold standard used to diagnose coronary artery disease. If a stress test identifies a problem with lack of blood flow to specific regions of the heart, the cardiologist may opt to treat a patient with medications. However, if the symptoms do not improve or if the stress test results show major ischemic changes, a more aggressive approach is necessary, and cardiac catheterization is done. When the patient develops acute coronary syndrome (ACS), a heart attack is imminent. In such a case, cardiac catheterization is often the next step to identify the culprit lesion causing coronary obstruction.

This test is done in a catheterization laboratory equipped with an X-ray machine and monitor screens set above a movable operating table. Oxygen and resuscitation equipment are available in case cardiac arrest occurs. The room is a sterile environment, much like a surgical suite, to prevent infections from occurring during cardiac procedures. The X-ray monitor shows the position of the heart and catheters and devices placed in the heart. Other monitors display pressure tracings from various blood vessels and from within the heart itself. A control room contains duplicate monitors and digital computer equipment that allows cardiac technologists to follow and record the entire procedure.

The patient is given a general sedative about an hour before the procedure and a local anesthetic is injected at the site of access. The patient is awake during the procedure so that he can report symptoms and follow directions for breath holding, coughing, and other maneuvers. Access to the heart is through a vein or artery in the arm or the groin. A wide-bore needle is placed in the blood vessel through a skin puncture, and a flexible plastic catheter (a hollow tube) inserted through the needle into the artery or the vein until it reaches the heart. The catheters are connected to pressure transducers that convert the physical pressures measured into electrical signals that can be displayed on a screen and recorded. When the catheter is passed through a vein, it passes through the right side of the heart and enters the left atrium, the left ventricle, and the pulmonary artery. As it traverses these regions, internal blood pressure readings can be recorded inside the heart and in the pulmonary circulation. These pressure readings are useful in making a diagnosis when there is ventricular dysfunction, valvular disease, and pulmonary hypertension and congenital heart disease. In some cases, a special cutting blade at the catheter tip is used to take a myocardial biopsy to make a diagnosis in cases of suspected hypertrophic cardiomyopathy, amyloidosis, and hemochromatosis.

If the catheter is inserted through an artery, it passes retrograde into the aorta, and then into the left ventricle through the aortic valve. Blood pressure in the aorta and left ventricle can be measured directly to determine if there is a gradient across the valve if there is aortic stenosis. Once the catheter is inside the left ventricle of the heart, dye is injected into the heart and rapid cine-photography done to show how the ventricle contracts. The radio-opaque dye outlines the shape of the ventricle. Playback of the images shows whether the heart is enlarged, whether it is pumping normally, or if there is valve leakage. This test is called a *ventriculogram*, and it is an excellent tool to show wall motion abnormalities if the person has an old scar from a myocardial infarction or a cardiomyopathy. This study is also useful in measuring end-diastolic and end-systolic volumes and for calculating the ejection fraction. These measurements provide reliable estimates of cardiac mechanical function as discussed earlier.

The catheter can also be positioned at the opening of the coronary arteries and radiographic dye injected directly into the artery. Since the dye is opaque to X-rays, the artery is visualized as it fills with dye. This procedure is called *arteriography* or *angiography*, and it is used to visualize arteries anywhere in the body. If there is a blockage, the artery is narrowed at the site and the extent of the problem can be identified. This study is essential to make a decision to perform angioplasty or coronary bypass surgery.

Generally, an artery needs to be blocked more than 70 percent before flow through it is seriously decreased. Partial blockages may actually cause no symptoms of chest pain. The reason that patients can often tolerate coronary artery blockages is that subsidiary channels open up around the blockage, called *collateral channels*, that provide blood to heart muscle. These collateral vessels can also be seen on coronary angiography as they ramify throughout the ventricular muscle. Though computed tomography (CT) scans are now being done as a noninvasive test for coronary artery disease, coronary angiography is still the gold standard for evaluating the coronary arteries.

Angioplasty, stenting, and other corrective and treatment procedures for atrial and ventricular septal defects can also be done during cardiac catheterization. Catheterization procedures generally take from about 1.5 hours for a catheterization that involves left and right heart catheterization and coronary angiography to 2–3 hours if angioplasty or other therapeutic procedures are also done.

Complications include tears caused in the arteries and veins by trauma from the catheters, and perforation of the heart walls with bleeding into the pericardium. Bleeding into the abdomen from the puncture of the groin artery or vein may occur, sometimes with the loss of considerable amounts of blood. Infection occurs rarely at the site of the arterial or venous puncture. Rarely, cardiac arrest and death can occur due to cardiac arrhythmias. Death from catheterization is rare, and this procedure is generally safe in experienced hands.

Radiological Studies of the Heart

Chest Radiography and Fluoroscopy

Chest radiography was the first radiologic test available to cardiologists after Wilhelm Roentgen (1845–1923) invented radiography, or X-ray imaging. Roentgen discovered X-rays in 1895 and won the first Nobel Prize in Physics in 1901. The technical term for an X-ray image is a *radiograph*. It is conventional to get a routine chest radiograph in all cases where heart disease is suspected. The heart becomes enlarged if there are problems with heart muscle function or if there is a hole in the heart from congenital heart disease. The heart is also enlarged in congestive heart failure. In the latter instance, the lungs appear translucent as fluid accumulates in the lung tissue. If a great deal of fluid accumulates, this appears as a dense white area that obliterates the transparent lung tissue, which is ordinarily filled with air. Such an accumulation is called a *pleural effusion*.

A modification of the chest X-ray is *fluoroscopy*, where the X-ray machine is left on and the movement of the heart seen on a TV monitor. With a continuous X-ray beam the heart can be seen beating and its shape and action discerned, while the lungs can be seen inflating and deflating. Movements of the diaphragm can also be seen. Fluoroscopy by itself is not done much these days, as much more sophisticated tests are available. Today fluoroscopy is done mostly in conjunction with cardiac catheterization and electrophysiological testing to determine where catheters should be placed within the heart. This method is used to guide cardiac interventions in real time, such as during angioplasty, electrophysiological studies, and pacemaker insertion.

Computed Tomography Scans

It is said that when Electrical and Musical Industries (EMI) supported the research of Godfrey Hounsfield (1919–2004), an engineer in England, they could afford it because of the money generated by the Beatles in the 1960s and 1970s. Subsequently, Hounsfield and Alan MacLeod Cormack (1924–1998), a physicist from Tufts University in Massachusetts, won the Nobel Prize in 1979 for their invention of computer tomography.

The word *tomography* means to "write in slices" (from the Greek *tomos*, meaning "slice"). A computerized tomogram is made by low-intensity X-rays that are delivered by a doughnut-shaped machine in a fan-like beam and recorded by a banana-shaped detector mounted on the opposite side. To make a CT of the head, the patient's head is placed inside the doughnut. The X-ray tube and the detector make a full 360-degree rotation around the head, so that images are made successively. The operation is computerized and the data fed into another image processing computer that creates slices that "see" the brain in different sections. This means that one view may be horizontally at the level of the fore-head, another at the level of the eye, another at the level of the nose, and so on. When viewed together in sequence, the technique provides a composite view of the brain by integrating the different slices. In some cases, it may be necessary to inject dye into a vein to outline blood vessels. The dye diffuses in one to two minutes and rapid CT images are made to outline the arteries and veins. This technique is called CT angiography, and injection of the dye is the only invasive part of the procedure. If there is a tumor, the blood supply to the tumor can also be seen. This method can also be applied to study the heart and the coronary arteries.

A new method of spiral CT can integrate the images into three-dimensions (3-D) using a computer. Actually, it is still a 2-D image but shaded and colored so that it looks like a real 3-D object and not a "slice" through the heart. This method actually shows the shape and size of the heart, the great arteries, and the coronary arteries. An estimate of narrowing or blockages of the coronary arteries can also be made, but a definitive diagnosis needs coronary angiography.

The risks of a CT scan include radiation exposure and allergic reactions to the dye. The total radiation from a CT-scan is not negligible and is equivalent to about a cumulative three- to five-year exposure to background radiation that we all receive normally. Allergic reactions to the dye are rare and may consist of rash, anaphylactic shock with cardiac arrest, and kidney damage.

Electron Beam Computed Tomography

This test is a special type of CT scan developed especially to study the human heart. It differs from conventional CT in that the electron beam is electronically spun in a circular fashion around the target. This method allows a very fast cir-cuit to be made around the heart, unlike a conventional CT that is mechanically spun around the target. The advantage is that electron beam computed tomogra-phy (EBCT) can image the beating heart quickly. However, it is a larger device and twice as expensive as a conventional CT.

This test is used to measure the calcium score of the coronary arteries. The calcium scan allegedly is a method to determine whether someone has coronary artery disease. The study measures the amount of calcium embedded in the walls of coronary arteries. A score is calculated for each coronary artery and a report generated. It is unclear how this test aids in the diagnosis of coronary artery disease, as much better functional and imaging tests such as stress testing and echocardiography are available. Currently, EBCT is largely promoted by radiologists who claim this test "screens" for asymptomatic coronary disease. Many people who take the test may be unnecessarily frightened if large amounts of calcium are discovered on the scan. It should be noted that most insurance plans do not pay for this test as it has not been definitively proven to be of value. In the opinion of many cardiologists, this method is largely a technology looking for a clinical application. It is possible that in the future, this test will be useful in the early detection of CAD.

Magnetic Resonance Imaging

Magnetic resonance imaging (MRI) does not use ionizing radiation like X-rays or CT scans. It is very recent in its use and the first human images were published in 1977. It is only fairly recently that decent images of organ structures could be obtained. In the past, it was difficult to obtain clear images of the heart as the heart moves constantly with each heartbeat. For an image to be made by MRI, the study organ has to be stationary. However, using gating techniques, it is now possible to obtain clear images of the heart and to make diagnoses of congenital heart disease, muscle disease, and tumors.

The technique uses powerful magnetic fields that involve the nuclear magnetization of hydrogen atoms in water contained in the body. Radiofrequency fields are then used to alter the alignment of the magnetized atoms. The changes in the magnetic fields are manipulated electronically to generate an image. In some ways cardiac MRI may be better than CT, but each has different uses and the doctor has to select the proper method for diagnosis. The main difference is that MRI does not expose the patient to radiation, and so can be used repeatedly to study disease conditions. However, in most cases, echocardiography and CT scanning are sufficient for diagnosis of most heart conditions and somewhat less expensive.

SUMMARY

Diagnosis of heart disease draws on a large variety of expensive tests, but in most cases it is not necessary to use all of the tests described above. There is a logical sequence from noninvasive to invasive tests, unless there is an emergency that requires urgent attention. Usually, an EKG and chest X-ray are done first. If there is chest pain or discomfort, the patient gets a stress test. If this test shows abnormalities, a cardiac catheterization is done if it is indicated, to look for blockages in the coronary arteries. The patient is then treated with medication, angioplasty, or surgery.

In the early stages of a myocardial infarction or if the person is having acute chest pains, it is unwise to do a stress test. In such cases, an EKG is done first and if there are acute changes suggesting a myocardial infarction is imminent, the patient is wheeled directly into a catheterization laboratory and invasive testing is done to reveal blockages in the coronary system. Treatments such as angioplasty and stenting can be done right away to correct the problem.

If there is an arrhythmia, and if it is considered serious, electrophysiological testing is done. A decision is then made whether a pacemaker or an implantable defibrillator is needed.

9

External and Implantable Cardiac Devices

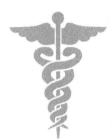

This chapter will describe the array of instruments and devices that are used to correct defective mechanical or electrical functions of the heart.

Implantable devices are generally deployed by cardiologists rather than by surgeons, except in remote areas where there are no cardiologists, but surgical care is available. The procedures are done in the catheterization suite under sterile conditions similar to the operating room. In the case of temporary transvenous cardiac pacing, the pacing electrode is inserted at the bedside in using sterile technique, as only a vein needs to be entered to deploy the catheter to the heart. Often, only light sedation is used and general anesthesia is not necessary in most cases. Broad-spectrum antibiotics are often administered before the procedure for implanted devices to avoid infection, though pretreatment is not always necessary.

The two broad categories of cardiac devices to correct either mechanical or electrical malfunction are listed below. Electronic devices are outlined in Table 9.1, and Table 9.2 shows the mechanical devices that are available, along with their respective functions.

Table 9.1 Implantable electronic devices and their functions

Electronic Device	What It Does
Electronic pacemaker	Discharges tiny bursts of electrical energy to make the heart beat regularly
Implantable cardioverter-defibrillator (ICD)	Delivers large burst of electricity to shock the heart out of a life-threatening arrhythmia (ventricular tachycardia or fibrillation)
Cardiac resynchronization device (CRD)	Paces the heart to improve electrical conduction patterns and contraction of the left ventricle

Table 9.2 Implantable mechanical cardiac devices and their functions

Mechanical Device	What It Does
Artificial heart	Replaces the normal heart and pumps blood and is used as a bridge to transplantation
Ventricular assist device (VAD)	Assists the heart when the left ventricle is damaged and used as a bridge to transplantation
Artificial valve	Allows one-way flow of blood when native valve is damaged, narrowed, or leaky
Septal occluder	Closes a hole in the heart to prevent blood shunting from one chamber into the adjacent chamber
Stent	Props open arteries to allow blood to flow freely

GENERAL CONSIDERATIONS

Cardiac electronic and pumping devices employ digital electrical circuitry containing programmable computer chips that control device functionality. The chips are factory-programmed, but the settings can be altered after implantation with special handheld devices that reset the rate, pulse duration, impulse current strength, and so forth. Miniaturization, with the use of printed circuit boards and transistors, has made electronic devices small enough so that they can be worn comfortably externally or implanted in the body. Such devices are powered by sealed lithium-iodide or similar batteries that last for 10 years or more, making replacement infrequent.

Pacemakers and implantable cardioverter-defibrillators (ICD), described below, contain memory chips that record and store the electrocardiogram (EKG). These devices can record and store abnormal rhythms that can be reviewed at a later time to make a diagnosis. In addition, ICDs contain a capacitor that charges up and stores electricity so that it can be discharged to treat cardiac arrhythmias, should the need arise. The arrhythmia being treated and the characteristics of the electrical discharge (shock strength, number of shocks, and the type of arrhythmia) are recorded and can be later printed out as a hard copy.

As the heart's electrical system ages, the normal cardiac pacemaker slows down and the heart rate becomes slower and slower. Sometimes the intrinsic sinoatrial (SA) node pacemaker beats at such a slow rate that it causes weakness, dizziness, or fainting. *Artificial pacemakers* help address this condition by regulating the heart rate to a more normal range.

A second kind of device is the *implantable cardioverter-defibrillator*. This device is implanted into patients who are resuscitated from sudden death caused by ventricular fibrillation, or those deemed to be at high risk for such death. Most ICDs provide artificial pacemaker functionality as well.

Mechanical failure of the heart leads to *congestive heart failure* or *pump failure*. Certain kinds of pacemakers are inserted that improve pumping action of the heart to treat pump failure. Pump failure often occurs in hearts that are badly scarred. Such hearts often have conduction abnormalities. This situation leads to asynchronous contraction of the ventricles due to delayed conduction of the cardiac impulse, so that cardiac efficiency is impaired. Implantation of a special pacemaker to restore a more normal conduction pattern synchronizes ventricular contraction and improves cardiac output to help relieve congestive heart failure.

Normal function of a device can be checked with an external monitoring device that, when placed on the skin over the implanted pacemaker, will record and transmit the EKG over a telephone line. Using this method, the rate of the device and other critical functions can be examined. If the battery runs down, the pulse rate will decline and a new generator needs to be implanted. This procedure is done in the catheterization laboratory under fluoroscopic guidance with conscious sedation in the same manner as the original implantation. If the patient dies, the pacemaker or ICD is often removed, especially if cremation is being considered.

Two other implanted devices that improve pumping action of the heart will be described later. The first is a left ventricular assist device (LVAD) and the second is an artificial heart. In addition, there are other smaller implantable devices that are purely mechanical (e.g., valves and venous filters), whose functions are to regulate the flow of blood and to prevent clots from traveling to the lungs.

PACEMAKERS AND WHAT THEY DO

The natural pacemaker of the heart slows down with age so that it may beat significantly below the normal rate of 60 beats per minute (bpm). In some cases, aging of the heart, or diseases like Lyme disease cause the heartbeat to slow down to the point that some beats do not actually reach the ventricles. This blockage occurs in the junction between the atria and the ventricles at the atrioventricular (AV) node. This is called *heart block*, an electrical phenomenon that slows down or prevents impulses from traveling from one part of the heart to another.

Like many other terms in medicine, the term *heart block* is sometimes misunderstood. While the term *block* suggests a *physical* impediment, this is not the case at all in heart block. The "block" in this case is actually an electrical block in impulses conducted within the electrical conduction system that connect the atria to the ventricles and make the heart beat in a synchronized manner. When the heartbeat slows down below 40 bpm in the waking state, the person becomes sluggish and tired, so much so that thinking and memory are impaired. If the heartbeat slows even further, there will be dizziness and fainting. Occasionally, there is a "pause" in the heartbeat and if it lasts for about 10–15 seconds, fainting occurs. In most cases, the heartbeat resumes spontaneously and the person recovers. An electrocardiogram often does not reveal anything more than a slow rate, as the actual period of heart block showing the prolonged pause may or may not occur during the time the EKG is recorded. Holter or telemetry monitoring will uncover this problem and a diagnosis can be easily made so that a pacemaker can be implanted.

Pacemakers were invented to normalize the heart rate when it slows to levels that cause symptoms. The older models were large battery packs that powered a pulse generator and an electrode. The pack is strapped to the patient and the electrode inserted through a vein and threaded into the heart. Today, the pulse generator is a unit that is smaller than a standard cell phone. It is fitted within a hermetically sealed titanium case with connections for the leads that contain the pacing electrodes at the tips. Figure 9.1 shows three types of implanted pacemaker.

These units are implanted under the skin below the collarbone and connected to the heart via a thin long cable electrode threaded into the subclavian vein, which is below the clavicle or collarbone. In early pacemakers, there was only one electrode and it was passed into the right ventricle through the tricuspid

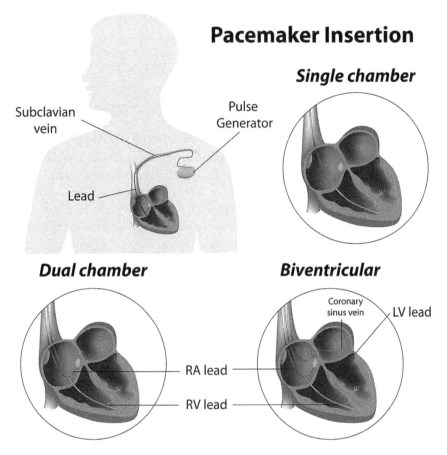

Figure 9.1 Three types of pacemakers used clinically. See text for details. © Alila07/ Dreamstime.com.

valve and wedged deep in the right ventricle (Figure 9.1 upper panel). Initially, in these older models, the pacemaker firing rate was fixed (e.g., at 60 pulses per minute [ppm]). When the heart rate slowed below 60 beats per minute, the pacemaker would kick in and take over pulsing the heart at a fixed rate of 60 ppm. Such fixed rate pacemakers are not ideal, as they cannot respond to physiological requirements (e.g., the need to increase rate with exercise or decrease it during sleep). Pacemakers that respond to exercise by sensing pectoral muscle activity using piezoelectric sensors were developed, so that cardiac output could be increased when the person is physically active. These devices are called *rate responsive pacemakers*.

Depending on the kind of pacemaker used and the purpose for which it was placed, there may be more than one electrode placed inside the heart. Ventricular pacing alone (single chamber pacing) is not physiological because the atria and ventricles are not synchronized to beat sequentially. Normally, the atria provide about 30 percent more blood to the ventricles when the two chambers work in sequence. To mimic the physiological sequence of a two-stage pump, a second electrode is placed in the right atrium. In this system, the atrium is paced first, and then a few milliseconds later the ventricle is stimulated by the pacemaker. This dual-lead system pacemaker is called an atrioventricular (AV) *dual chamber pacemaker* (Figure 9.1 lower left panel). This type of AV sequential pacemaker is considered more physiologically accurate as it mirrors normal heart activation and it boosts cardiac output when compared to ventricular pacing alone.

A third kind of pacing is used with patients suffering from congestive heart failure who do not improve with medications alone. When the heart is damaged and scarred, not only is the stroke volume lowered, but there are also abnormalities in how the electrical impulse travels within the conduction system of the heart. There is a delay in the way the two ventricles are activated so that there is slightly asynchronous pumping action. This situation leads to abnormal contraction patterns of the left ventricle resulting in a lack of coordination between the two pumping chambers. To normalize the contraction pattern, one lead is placed in the right ventricle and the other in the coronary sinus vein to activate the left ventricle (Figure 9.1 lower right panel). These pacemakers reconfigure the ventricular activation sequence to make it more normal and provide *cardiac resynchronization therapy* (CRT). This small correction in ventricular activation is enough to boost cardiac output and help improve symptoms of congestive heart failure in about 70 percent of cases. In selected patients, CRT improves quality of life, functional status, and exercise capacity. Survival is also improved in these cases even if a defibrillator is not implanted.

Not all patients are suitable for CRT, as they have to meet certain clinical and EKG criteria that suggest this treatment will be beneficial. Though CRT is expensive, preliminary data show that all-cause mortality and all-cause hospitalizations are reduced by this treatment. In the long run, it may actually be cost-saving to use CRT in selected patients who qualify for this treatment.

EXTERNAL TEMPORARY PACING OF THE HEART

Temporary pacing may be necessary in patients awaiting permanent pacing or when temporary damage to the conduction system occurs. When a permanent pacer cannot be immediately inserted, a temporary electrode is placed in the heart through a vein and connected to an external pacemaker. Some patients in remote areas without a cardiologist or a surgeon who can install a permanent pacemaker require temporary pacing before being transported to another hospital for such treatment. In other patients, especially following acute inferior myocardial infarction, there may be reversible heart block that requires only temporary pacing with an external pacemaker.

There are also external pacemakers that do not have electrodes inserted into the heart. Such pacemakers do not require any special skills to be used as they are completely external and can be used by nurses and emergency medical technicians. These pacers are attached to the chest with large, flat adhesive electrodes placed over the heart, and they stimulate the heart through the chest wall. This procedure is used for standby pacing in relatively stable patients as a precautionary step when the heart rate is slow as heart block may occur in such patients. Though it does not require an invasive procedure, the chest may twitch uncomfortably if the output current is too high. This approach is ideal in situations where there is no expertise available to insert an electrode into the heart in order to provide direct temporary pacing.

Temporary pacing is often utilized during open-heart surgery. In this situation, electrode leads are sutured onto the surface of the heart for external (epicardial) pacing during open chest surgery, as there may be inadvertent damage to the conduction system. Trauma to the heart during cardiac surgery occasionally leads to very slow heart rates or heart block. Often, these problems resolve several days after surgery and the wires are then pulled out through the skin when they are no longer needed. In rare instances, a permanent pacemaker needs to be implanted if the problem does not resolve spontaneously several days after surgery, and heart block persists.

IMPLANTABLE CARDIOVERTER-DEFIBRILLATORS

An implantable cardioverter-defibrillator (ICD) is like a pacemaker, but built into the generator is a capacitor that stores electrical energy. In the simplest configuration, the defibrillator electrode lead is placed much like a pacing electrode in the right ventricle. If pacing is required, another electrode is often placed in the right atrium. The sensing electrode feeds signals from the heart and when the ICD detects that ventricular fibrillation has occurred, it automatically discharges a burst of current delivered via the defibrillator electrodes. If normal rhythm is not restored, the defibrillator discharges again and again until it detects a normal rhythm.

The ICD can be interrogated by using an external probe placed over the ICD itself connected to a machine that can read the information stored in the computer chip inside the device. The ICD can store EKGs and information such as heart rate, the rhythms, detected the discharges of the device (if any), and the timing of these events in its memory chip. This provides useful information on the heart's activity, especially if a bout of arrhythmia occurred and if the device was activated by this event. This information is used to tailor appropriate treatment and adjust the sensitivity and settings of the ICD device as required.

Patients who have been resuscitated from cardiac arrest due to ventricular fibrillation are likely to face another cardiac arrest. Strangely, it is people with coronary artery disease who had cardiac arrest without any damage to the heart muscle who are particularly liable to have recurrent ventricular fibrillation. This group, which accounts for two-thirds of all patients with cardiac arrest, requires special protection against ventricular fibrillation with drugs or an ICD or both.

Oddly enough, if cardiac arrest occurs during a myocardial infarction, ventricular fibrillation does not tend to recur. In such people, the long-term outlook is much the same as in someone who has not had a cardiac arrest, especially if left ventricular function is preserved. However, those patients with an ejection fraction less than 30–35 percent are considered to be at high risk for sudden death. Many cardiac specialists believe that, based on current data, ICD treatment is superior to drug treatment for serious ventricular arrhythmias in reducing cardiac mortality in these patients.

Once implanted, these devices need to be monitored in the outpatient clinic every 4–6 months for battery life and proper functioning. At the end of life of the battery, more frequent monitoring is necessary. Untoward discharge of the device will need evaluation and if lead fracture is present, replacement of the electrode is necessary.

ARTIFICIAL HEARTS AND VENTRICULAR ASSIST DEVICES

When there is severe loss of cardiac muscle (e.g., in very advanced left ventricular dysfunction in cardiomyopathy or after myocardial infarction), heart function may not improve with medications or pacemaker therapy. In such cases the only good option is a heart transplant. Since there is a severe shortage of donor hearts, two types of devices exist that can buy time: an artificial heart and a ventricular assist device (VAD).

The total artificial heart is made by SynCardia Systems, Inc. (Tucson, Arizona) and was approved by the Food and Drug Administration in 2004 after 10 years of experimentation. Since then over 1,000 implantations have been performed so far. Another artificial heart is produced by Abiomed, Inc. (Danvers, Massachusetts) and is totally implantable, including the power supply. However, because of the large size of the heart itself and the large battery pack, it cannot be implanted in most women and many men who have smaller chest cavity size. As of 2009, the heart has been implanted 14 times and none of the patients are still alive. This type of heart is no longer actively in use currently. Artificial heart implantation is not a permanent solution as there are still significant problems with power supply, infection, blood clotting, and other long-term problems. An artificial heart is either a "bridge" to a transplant, or "destination" therapy as a permanent solution if a biological heart is not available.

Ventricular assist devices (VAD), also called left ventricular assist devices (LVAD), are another bridging device for heart transplantation. When the left ventricle is severely damaged, its function can be assisted by a battery-powered mechanical pump that is surgically implanted in the upper abdomen on the left side. It receives blood from the left ventricle and pumps it into the aorta so that circulation is maintained. The LVAD is connected to an externally worn control unit and battery. With this procedure, patients can be discharged and sent home to await transplantation. Former Vice President Dick Cheney received such a device in 2010 and ultimately received a heart transplant in early 2012 at the age of 71. It has been shown that such pumps reduce death rates by about 50 percent over the course of a year and also extends life.

OTHER MECHANICAL DEVICES

The other mechanical devices such as stents, artificial valves, and septal closure devices are discussed in more detail in other sections in this book (see Chapters 3, 4, and 7).

COMPLICATIONS

Implantation of devices such as pacemakers, ICDs, LVADs, and valves may result in either infection or bleeding. In both cases, the consequences may be serious and will need to be treated appropriately. Sterile technique and careful attention to control of bleeding are therefore essential. Implantation of pacemakers and ICDs is done below the right or left clavicle and the electrodes are inserted transvenously (i.e., through a large vein leading to the heart). Occasionally, the lung is entered accidentally and a pneumothorax (collapsed lung) results. If the pneumothorax is large, the complication requires treatment by inserting a lung tube to drain air.

Before implantation is performed, sedation is administered and antibiotics are given to reduce the chance of infection. If infection does occur, the device has to be removed and the infected site treated before re-implantation can be done.

Bleeding may occur, as the skin is breached and the vein is entered, with accumulation of blood into the chest cavity. Rarely, an electrode may pierce the wall of the heart and bleeding may occur into the pericardium. This may require removal of the blood with a needle to avoid complications arising from the heart being squeezed, to the extent that blood pressure declines, and the patient goes into shock. This condition is called *pericardial tamponade* and can sometimes lead to death if it is left untreated. Electrode leads may also fracture, in which case the function of the device will be rendered ineffective.

Very rarely, the pacemaker may fire rapidly and inappropriately, resulting in a condition called *runaway pacemaker*. An ICD may discharge inappropriately and randomly. Placing a doughnut-hole magnet over the device will result in the pacemaker going into a *fixed rate mode*. This means the device when activated by the magnet adopts a default setting and starts to pulse at a fixed rate regardless of the need for pacing. This move allows for diagnostics to be performed and the device reprogrammed or replaced if necessary. If an ICD fires repeatedly and inappropriately, it can also be deactivated in a similar manner, simply by taping a magnet over the pacemaker until it is replaced.

Pacemakers and ICDs may occasionally suffer interference by other types of magnets, like those found in headphones for MP3 players (e.g., iPods), some types of heavy machinery, and electric motors. Microwaves may also interfere with the devices and make them malfunction. However, despite this possibility, most electrical devices, electric blankets, MP3 players, cell phones, metal detectors, and handheld airport security scans do not interfere with normal function if they are not too close to the device.

ETHICAL AND LEGAL ISSUES

The interaction between humans and life-sustaining medical devices has created a new set of ethical and legal dilemmas. There are several related issues: the quality of life of the person, the cost of the treatment to the person and to society, and the wishes of the person. Even if the person is sapient and can make an informed decision, it is often very difficult for a person to arrive at a decision if it means ending one's own life. The complexity is increased when factoring in competing opinions of doctors, and the different stakes that each caregiver and relative hold. Religious beliefs, as well as social status and political clout, also play a role in this decision making.

While there is legal precedent for withdrawing care in critically ill patients to allow them to die, there is less certainty about what to do with pacemakers, ICDs, VADs, and artificial hearts in conscious patients. If the patient is unconscious, semiconscious and mentally incompetent, or has experienced severe brain damage, the decision is much easier, as the devices can be turned off after notification of family members assuming there is consensus among them and the team. For pacemakers, these devices are generally left on until death occurs first. In the case of ICD, it is generally agreed that the person will not be given CPR and the device is turned off so it doesn't fire and attempt to revive the heart. The guidelines are thus the same as for a *do-not-resuscitate* (DNR) order with external defibrillation not being permitted.

In the case of VAD and artificial hearts, the decision is more complex and discussions among caregivers, the patient, and the family are needed to make a final determination. Rarely, the state is involved and a legal opinion may be required. To date, no successful litigation has occurred in artificial heart implantation when patients have not survived, probably because families recognize the dire nature of the illness and the heroic measures already undertaken by a dedicated team.

SUMMARY

With the invention of circuit boards and transistors, the miniaturization of electronic devices made it possible to create small devices that can be implanted in the body. These advances made it possible to create small implantable pacemakers and ICDs that extend life. Mechanical devices are also available to assist left ventricular function to improve circulation and as a bridge to cardiac transplantation. Other devices help improve valvular function and close congenital heart defects. With many life-sustaining devices, the decision to withdraw care has become a matter for legal and ethical debate.

10

Surgical Treatment for Heart Disease

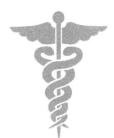

Case Study

An 80-year-old Orthodox rabbi from New York City was seen in Boston for consultation for aortic stenosis. His cardiologist discovered a harsh cardiac murmur when he complained of shortness of breath and dizziness on exertion. An echocardiogram showed a large gradient across the aortic valve suggesting severe aortic stenosis. His cardiologist recommended valve replacement as the rabbi had mild symptoms. In a second consultation, another cardiologist in New York agreed that the rabbi needed cardiac catheterization and probable valve replacement. The rabbi sought a third opinion in Boston because he was troubled and thought that, "Everyone thinks I should have surgery." According to him, Jewish law and tradition required that at least one person should dissent, so that there is a fair arbitration with presentation of both sides of the case. When I saw him, I recommended that he have cardiac catheterization to determine the degree of aortic stenosis.

He agreed to return to Boston for cardiac catheterization, and the study revealed a gradient of 65 millimeters across the aortic valve. The coronary arteries were normal and the left ventricle was thickened, but contraction was normal. I recommended a porcine valve replacement because of his age and as this would not require anticoagulation with a blood thinner. He called his rabbi in Jerusalem who told him to go ahead with surgery. He was relieved to hear that Jewish law did not proscribe a pig valve because it did not violate dietary restrictions. The aortic valve was successfully replaced thorough an open chest procedure and he recovered without complications.

Surgery is the treatment of diseases or injuries with physical interventions using specialized techniques and instruments. The term *surgery* comes from the Latin *chirurgiae*, which translates roughly as "to work by hand." Healers have practiced surgery for thousands of years in Greek, Persian, Tibetan, Chinese, and Indian cultures by devising and using surgical instruments, sutures, casts, and other devices. Today, operative procedures are done in a specially equipped operating room or OR (known as an *operating theatre*, or OT, in British English). Procedures in cardiology that do not fall under the rubric of *surgery* are procedures such as cardiac catheterization, angioplasty, or the placement of stents and cardiac devices within the heart or blood vessels. These procedures are called *invasive* or *interventional procedures*.

Modern surgery had its beginnings in times of war, especially after guns became commonplace in the 1400s and field surgeons had to treat major injuries on the battlefield. The practice of modern surgery is attributed to Ambroise Paré (1510–1590), who famously said *"Je le pansai, Dieu le guérit"* ("I apply the dressing and God heals the wound"). He abandoned the common practice of applying hot oil to wounds and instead used an ointment of egg yolk and turpentine that promoted healing. Paré also introduced the concept of tying off of arteries (ligation) with sutures to control bleeding, instead of cauterization with a red-hot iron.

Three major advances led to the development of successful modern surgery: sterile surgical techniques, anesthesia, and blood transfusions. Infection was once the leading cause of sickness and death during the postoperative recovery phase. It was the introduction of sterile techniques during surgery by Joseph Lister (1827–1912) in 1867 that led to our understanding of antisepsis. This approach substantially decreased wound infection following surgery. Until the discovery, around 1865, that bacteria could cause wound putrefaction and other undesirable effects by the French bacteriologist Louis Pasteur (1822–1895), the actual cause of infections was not known. Along with Robert Koch (1843–1910) in Germany, Pasteur was responsible for the germ theory of disease. The discovery of antibiotics in the first part of the 20th century further helped to stifle infections that inadvertently sometimes occur despite sterile surgery.

Second, the development of surgical anesthesia allowed all kinds of major and minor surgical procedures to be done with a high degree of safety. Longer and more complex operations were possible and better tolerated because of anesthesia as the patient was unaware of the pain and could not disrupt the surgical procedure. Though alcohol, opium, and nitrous oxide were used for dulling pain during dental and surgical procedures, the first real anesthetic was ether. Ether anesthesia was officially introduced to medical practitioners by William T.G. Morton (1819–1868). He never graduated from either the Baltimore College of Dental Surgery or Harvard Medical School, both of which he attended, but this did not prevent him from practicing dentistry.

In 1846, Morton successfully administered ether at the Massachusetts General Hospital in Boston, where John Collins Warren (1778–1856), the first dean at Harvard Medical School, removed a tumor from the neck of Edward G. Abbott. After the successful operation, of which the patient had no recollection, Warren famously said, "Gentlemen, this is no humbug." The operating room, now called the Ether Dome, is listed as a National Historic Monument of the United States. Morton published this event later that year, but Crawford Long (1815–1878), a Georgia physician, challenged Morton's claim as he claimed to have used ether four years earlier, in 1842. Chloroform was also used for surgical anesthesia by James Young Simpson (1811–1870), a Scottish obstetrician. It was found to cause cardiac arrhythmias, and chloroform was later abandoned in Europe in favor of ether.

Some operations inevitably resulted in massive amounts of blood loss, so it was necessary to devise a process for replacing that blood. The development of blood transfusion is vital so that the body maintains normal blood volume, perfusion, and oxygenation during surgery. In early experiments, blood was transfused from animals to humans, as well as between humans, but this was often not successful due to biological incompatibility. In 1901, Karl Landsteiner (1868–1943), an Austrian-born American physician, discovered the blood groups A, B, AB, and C (later called O). Blood transfusions between groups with different blood types causes the blood to clump due to immune incompatibility, and this can lead to death. Nowadays, blood from donors is typed according to Landsteiner's classification and subtyped for the Rh factor as well, and matched with the potential patient's blood type before surgery. Prior to surgery, the patient often contributes his own blood for himself, or the correct blood type has to be stocked, so that the surgeon can replace blood loss.

THE OPERATING ROOM

With the advent of hospitals in Europe in the late 17th century, doctors actually posed a threat to the health of patients as they often carried germs that caused infections. The germ theory was not known and doctors wore street clothes and operated on patients without gloves. Mothers delivering babies were at special risk for puerperal sepsis and death, as aseptic technique was not practiced.

In 1847, the Hungarian physician Ignaz Semmelweiss (1818–1865), while working in Vienna, showed that simple hand washing with a chlorinated lime solution significantly reduced deaths from puerperal sepsis following childbirth. He was met with fierce resistance when he tried to implement aseptic techniques in the maternity wards. In 1883, the German surgeon Gustav Neuber (1850–1932) introduced the concept of a separate sterile surgical suite with gowns, head and shoe covers for personnel, and the use of instruments sterilized in an autoclave. Before this time, death rates from infections during surgery ranged from 25–60 percent if the patient managed to survive the operation.

Today, surgical procedures are done in a sterile environment that is in a secure, limited-access area of a hospital or clinic. Surgical operation suites are specially engineered to minimize infections during surgery. Changing areas are provided to change from street clothes and shoes into fresh gowns and footwear. Sinks and antiseptic detergents are provided for scrubbing hands and arms prior to performing surgery. To further minimize bacterial contamination, operating rooms are equipped with ventilation from wall-mounted units providing unidirectional horizontal laminar flow of clean air from High-Efficiency Particulate Air (HEPA) filtration systems.

Even with these precautions, surgical site infections cause serious mortality and morbidity. Examples of life-threatening infections are "flesh-eating bacteria" (*Streptococcus pyogenes*) and methicillin-resistant *Staphylococcus aureus* (MRSA), which produce toxins that are fatal. Humans are the major source of infections postoperatively, with men carrying more germs than women. Therefore, all personnel who have contact with patients have to change into scrub suits and wear masks as well as head and beard covers. If they do not have special clogs for the OR, shoe covers are required as well.

All drapes and instruments coming in contact with a patient are sterilized prior to use. Following surgery, all equipment, including the table, intravenous poles, and so forth, are wiped clean with an antiseptic solution. Heavily infected cases are operated on in a dedicated OR. The entire room is fumigated by a special team before another patient is operated upon. These procedures are effective in reducing hospital-acquired infections by preventing patient-to-patient transmission of germs.

The OR is equipped with a raised movable operating table with strong overhead lighting, outlets in the wall for suction of blood and fluids, anesthetic gas outlets, and a cart with equipment for delivery of anesthetic gases and oxygen. There are also electrocardiogram and blood pressure monitoring equipment and infusion pumps to deliver medications as needed. A tray-table holds sterile instruments that the scrub nurse hands to the surgeon during the operation. A heart-lung machine for cardiopulmonary bypass pump is wheeled in if the heart is going to be stopped during surgery. Computers are used for tracking vital signs, blood gas levels, fluid and blood administration, and so forth. In some ORs there is radiographic imaging equipment such as X-ray machines, surgical robots, videoscopic units, ultrasound, computed tomography (CT), and magnetic resonance imaging (MRI) scanners to guide surgery and to determine if the surgeon has accomplished a favorable result before the patient leaves the OR.

PREPARATION FOR SURGERY

At least one day before the operation, the patient is evaluated by an anesthesiologist to ensure that the patient is fit enough to undergo surgery. This screening also helps determine if there are preoperative problems that need to be addressed. Such issues include mild congestive heart failure, electrolyte disorders, uncontrolled high blood pressure, uncontrolled diabetes, kidney disease, and bleeding problems. In older patients who may have carotid artery disease there may be a risk of a stroke or brain damage due to decreased blood flow to the brain. Carotid artery blood flow studies are needed to determine if surgery on a blocked carotid artery needs to be done before cardiac surgery is performed. This process reduces the chance of a stroke during or after surgery. In emergency cases, the surgeon obviously has less time, and more rapid screening is done.

The operating surgeon also evaluates the patient and reviews all tests, often well before surgery is performed, or just prior to surgery in emergencies. He obtains a signed consent for the procedure after explaining the risks and benefits of the intended surgery. In the Western world and many other countries, it is illegal to operate on a patient without *written informed consent*. Operating without written consent of the person in the United States is tantamount to assault and battery, and the surgeon can be sued for malpractice. If the patient is a minor or is mentally incompetent due to confusion, brain injury, or mental illness, the surgeon obtains written consent from a legal guardian, or with an appropriate adult present, or through a court order. In emergency situations, the surgeon or treating physician may utilize the legal principle of *executive privilege* to save the life of the patient, and written or verbal consent is not required. Legal prosecution is rare in such life-threatening cases.

THE OPERATIVE PROCEDURE

The goal of cardiac surgery is to correct the cardiac defect, while controlling excessive blood loss. Simultaneously, the surgeon and anesthesiologist have to ensure protection of the heart, brain, and kidneys in order to avoid cardiac damage, stroke, and kidney failure. The patient fasts overnight to empty the stomach. This is done so the patient does not vomit during or after surgery as this will cause a chemical inhalation pneumonia. The patient receives preoperative sedation to relax even before anesthesia is administered later in the operation suite.

Intravenous and arterial lines and a urinary catheter are inserted. An endotracheal tube is inserted into the throat, and anesthesia is then induced using anesthetic gases along with oxygen. The chest and any other operative field are shaved if necessary and cleansed with an antiseptic solution to avoid contamination by bacteria. Since the body is unclothed, the patient will need to be covered with sterile drapes exposing only the chest and the groin areas.

Sticky electrodes are placed on the skin to record the EKG. The arterial line is used to monitor blood pressure, and oxygen saturation of the blood is continuously monitored. These values are displayed on a computer monitor visible to both the surgeon and the anesthesiologist. It is necessary to make sure throughout the operation that blood pressure and oxygen saturation are maintained at levels that will prevent brain damage during surgery.

The skin is opened using a scalpel, and a bone-cutting electric saw is used to split the breastbone vertically to approach the heart from the front. The split sternum is held open with a special clamp to expose the heart. The tissue and fat around the heart are dissected to allow access to the heart so that surgery can be performed. Electrocautery equipment, consisting of a metal probe heated by electricity, is used to stop bleeding from small vessels. Large vessels are tied off using sutures.

The beating heart has to be stopped to do surgery for coronary artery bypass, repair of atrial or ventricular septal defects, and other congenital heart diseases. A heart-lung cardiopulmonary bypass (CPB) machine is used so that circulation can continue during surgery. The machine, developed by John H. Gibbon (1903–1973) and others, uses a mechanical pump and allows for circulation of oxygenated blood. In 1953, 18-year-old Cecelia Bavolek was operated on by Gibbon for an atrial septal defect, becoming the first person to successfully undergo open-heart surgery. For 26 minutes, which was more than half the duration of the operation, the machine totally supported her heart and lung functions.

The patient is placed on a CPB machine by placing a large bore cannula (tube) in the right atrium (to drain blood from the venous side), and another smaller catheter into the ascending aorta to return oxygenated blood to the body. The machine is primed with heparin to prevent blood from clotting as it is circulated. The aorta is cross-clamped and a cold solution rich in potassium is infused into the heart. As the solution is cold and toxic, it cools the heart and induces *cardioplegia,* or "paralysis of the heart." This solution causes the heart to stop beating. Hypothermia, the other key component of cardioplegia, protects the heart by lowering metabolism so that myocardial oxygen consumption is reduced by 95 percent. Cold cardioplegia allows the body to be maintained for up to 45 minutes without blood flow. Normally, permanent brain damage occurs in three to 4 minutes if there is no circulation. Inducing hypothermia and cold cardioplegia allows surgery to be performed for a couple of hours with a very low risk of brain damage.

In some heart operations CPB is not utilized and the chest is not even opened to expose the heart. The surgeon may perform "keyhole" or *minimally invasive surgery* (MIS) where holes are made between the ribs. In such cases, a video probe is inserted through one keyhole and the heart and the inside of the heart viewed on a TV monitor. Then, through two other keyholes, the surgeon enters the heart using scissors in one hand and forceps in the other, and performs the surgical procedure under indirect visual guidance. Suturing of cut structures or placement of a valve can be done with this method. The same procedure is used for removing a tumor inside the heart or for aortic and mitral valve repair or replacement. More recently, robots guided by the surgeon are used to perform such surgical procedures.

Often, during and after the surgical procedure, a transesophageal echocardiogram (TEE) is done. This allows the surgeon to see the heart's pumping action, the movement of the valves and the great vessels, and fluid in the pericardium. Doppler echocardiography shows blood flow patterns within the heart. The surgical result can thus be checked and modified in real time before the chest is closed.

On completion of the procedure, the surgeon ensures there are no bleeding points, and makes a thorough check that there are no instruments or sponges left behind inside the patient. Surgical trauma causes oozing of blood and plasma to occur inside the chest for many days afterwards. Drainage tubes attached to external suction pumps are placed in the chest so that oozing fluid and blood can be drained over the next few days. The body is rewarmed, if cooling has been initiated, the bypass pump disconnected, and all surgical clamps are removed from the heart and chest wall. When the heart is rewarmed, it restarts beating, often on its own, though sometimes electric shocks or pacing are needed to restart the heart. A final check is made for bleeding, sponges, and instruments, before the chest is closed. The split sternum is closed with steel wire sutures and the skin wound closed with silk sutures.

In open-chest heart operations, the surgeon sews pacemaker electrodes directly onto the heart and threads the wires through the skin before closing the chest. If it is needed, a pacemaker can be attached and switched on to keep the heart beating at a normal rate. If it is not needed postoperatively, the pacemaker wires are simply removed a few days after surgery by tugging them out through the chest wall.

CARDIAC SURGERY FOR SELECTED CONDITIONS

Coronary Bypass Surgery

Coronary artery bypass surgery (CABG, often pronounced as "cabbage") is a procedure that is done about 500,000 times a year in the United States. During this procedure a blockage in a coronary artery is bypassed by using another artery or a vein. The idea is to provide blood supply to the heart muscle by means other than opening up the blockage itself. There are several claims as to who did the first operation. Like many new inventions and procedures, several surgeons embarked on projects at about the same time, and exact precedence is sometimes difficult to determine.

In 1960 at the Albert Einstein College of Medicine, Robert Goetz and Michael Rohman, assisted by Jordan Haller and Ronald Dee, used the internal mammary artery to bypass a blockage of the right coronary artery. The internal mammary arteries run down each side of the sternum (breastbone). Usually the left mammary artery is used after it is freed from its usual position and then implanted onto the blocked coronary artery.

In 1962, at the Johns Hopkins University School of Medicine, David Sabiston (1924–2009) operated on a patient's beating heart and used a vein stripped from the patient's leg to bypass a blocked coronary artery. The patient later had a stroke and died. In 1964, Michael E. DeBakey (1908–2008) assisted by Edward Garrett did what is generally considered to be the first successful coronary bypass using a vein from the leg of the patient. This was made possible by improvements in the heart-lung machine.

René Gerónimo Favaloro (1923–2000), originally from Argentina, working at the Cleveland Clinic in 1967, started to consistently use the saphenous vein removed from the leg for the bypass grafting procedure. This vein is very long; it stretches from the ankle to the groin and may be 30–40 inches long in an adult. The vein can be cut into three or four pieces and used for multiple bypass grafts in the heart. This method for bypass grafting has become the standard technique today. Fewer operations are done using internal mammary arteries, often only in combination with venous bypass grafting.

The basic principle for CABG is that the vein graft or the mammary artery creates a detour around the blocked coronary artery to provide oxygenated blood to the heart muscle. The surgeon already knows the location of the coronary obstructive lesion by having screened the coronary angiogram. He can also locate the obstruction in the coronary artery by touch during surgery. The surgeon attaches the vein graft or mammary artery to the coronary artery just below the blockage. If a vein is used, the other end is attached to the root of the aorta, which becomes the source of blood supply (Figure 10.1). In most cases, between two to five coronary bypass grafts are done at the same time. Single vessel grafting is almost never performed as such blockages are best treated by angioplasty.

The success rate of CABG surgery in relieving angina is high, and about 90 percent of patients experience significant improvement in symptoms after surgery. Full relief from chest pain and resumption of normal activities occurs in about 70 percent of cases. The remaining patients experience partial relief from angina. In 5–10 percent of CABG surgery, the bypass graft becomes blocked by a clot or fibrotic scar tissue within one year. Patients who smoke, who have long-standing

Coronary artery bypass surgery

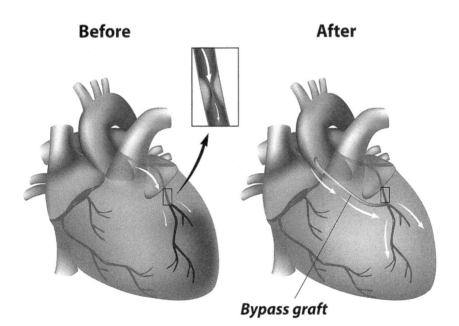

Before   **After**

Bypass graft

Figure 10.1 Coronary artery bypass surgery. The left panel shows the site of obstruction in the left anterior descending (LAD) coronary artery (in the inset). The right panel shows the bypass graft in place connecting the aorta to the LAD. © Alila07/Dreamstime.com.

insulin-dependent diabetes, and who are over 70 years are less likely to experience ideal results from CABG. It is therefore important for patients to stop smoking, to take care of their diet, weight, and cholesterol levels, and to exercise in order to fully benefit from surgery.

It may come as a surprise that CABG does not prolong life in all cases of CAD, even when all major obstructions are successfully treated with grafting. Bypass surgery for increasing survival is limited to a small subset of patients with CAD. In an American Heart Association conference of experts in 2011 chaired by L. David Hillis from the University of Texas, a consensus was agreed upon regarding patients who may have a survival benefit from CABG. These subsets include:

- Patients with left main coronary artery obstruction of 50 percent or more
- Significant obstruction (70% or more) of three major coronary arteries
- Significant obstruction of the left anterior coronary artery (LAD) and one other artery
- Significant obstruction of two major coronary arteries with extensive myocardial ischemia on stress testing
- Mild to moderate left ventricular dysfunction (35%–50% ejection fraction) and significant multivessel or proximal LAD disease

A detailed discussion of criteria agreed on by this conference can be found in the *Journal of the American College of Cardiology*, 58 (2011): 123–210.

Off-Pump Coronary Artery Bypass (OPCAB) surgery is a procedure in which the heart is not stopped completely during surgery, but greatly slowed by medications. The operating field over the heart where the coronary artery is located is held down and stabilized with special instruments. The heart is still beating slowly and the surgeon sews the graft in place between heartbeats. This method can only be used in a minority of patients, but it avoids use of the bypass machines, and hence may reduce complications.

More recently, the above technique has been used through a small incision in the front of the chest and without splitting the sternum. Minimally invasive coronary artery direct bypass (MIDCAB) surgery is sometimes done if the blocked artery is in the front of the heart and can be easily accessed by an incision between the ribs so that the chest is not opened. The ribs are separated and the left internal mammary artery used to bypass the blockage. This procedure is done without the bypass pump, as described previously.

A more refined form of such surgery is found with the totally endoscopic coronary artery bypass surgery (TECAB), developed in the late 1990s. The U.S. Department of Defense developed a novel concept to enable remote surgery (i.e., "in the field") to meet the needs of battlefield conditions and allow skilled on-site medics to work with surgeons at a central location. The idea was to have a fully equipped OR on wheels that could travel to the battlefield to treat wounded soldiers. The *da Vinci telerobotic surgery system* evolved from these and other academic and industrial efforts. The technique involves making three or four small holes in the chest cavity through which two robotic arms and a camera are inserted. This procedure utilizes a three-dimensional telerobotic imaging system made by Intuitive Surgical Inc., called the da Vinci surgical system.

The surgeon sits at an ergonomically designed computer console and views a three-dimensional virtual operative field through a binocular system. The visual field shows a virtual image of the operative site. The surgeon performs the operation by controlling four robotic arms, which hold the stereoscopic video camera and surgical instruments that mimic hand motions. The three-dimensional imaging and hand-like motions of the system facilitate advanced invasive thoracic, cardiac, and abdominal procedures (e.g., hysterectomy and prostate operations). In civilian life, the patient is on an operating table with the surgeon performing the operation in close proximity and not from a remote location.

For CABG-like procedures, the surgeon uses the robot to free the internal mammary artery and link it to a blocked coronary artery. In many cases, recovery is rapid and, barring any complications, the patient can be discharged the following day. This type of procedure reduces pain, shortens hospital stay, and allows for rapid recovery if there are no complications such as serious bleeding or infection. If complications occur during surgery, such as difficulty in completing the operation or bleeding, the surgeon has to open the chest and resort to more traditional methods.

It is important to realize that CABG is not done in order to save lives, but to relieve symptoms of angina, increase quality of life, and reduce disability. Such surgery does not prolong life, nor does angioplasty, in the majority of cases. However, surgery is successful in relieving angina more completely than angioplasty does and the results last longer. Even airline pilots can now return to their former work following successful cardiac surgery. Surgery is also the better procedure in complicated multivessel disease where angioplasty is difficult to perform. But before considering surgery for stable angina, it is best to first attempt treating a patient with medications and to implement lifestyle changes. Patients are encouraged to avoid smoking, reduce weight, control cholesterol and fat intake, and maintain an exercise program. If such treatment is unsuccessful, the patient and his doctor should consider a surgical option.

Valve Surgery

Diseases of the aortic and mitral valves are the most common conditions encountered in valvular disease. The aortic and mitral valves are affected by congenital defects or by rheumatic heart disease as a child, adolescent, or young adult. Young people may develop rheumatic fever following throat infections, resulting in narrowing of the mitral valve called mitral stenosis. Older people develop aortic stenosis (narrowing), aortic regurgitation (leaky valve), or mitral regurgitation due to calcium deposits or degeneration of the valve tissue.

In some cases, a narrowed mitral, pulmonic, or aortic valve can be cracked open by inflating a balloon catheter. This procedure is done by inserting a catheter with a balloon at its tip that is inflated when the catheter is threaded to the valve. The balloon tip is positioned exactly at the opening of the valve as guided by the X-ray fluoroscope monitor. Expansion of the balloon by injecting contrast material into the catheter will force open the valve leaflets and improve blood flow. Significant improvement in CHF can occur even when the gradient across the valve is reduced slightly. Though the valve may be damaged or torn during the procedure, it is optimal for older or very frail patients who may not be in any condition to undergo the trauma of open-heart surgery and valve replacement.

In the case of our patient described at the beginning of the chapter, though he was 80 years old, he was lean, fit, and had no other complicating illnesses. All these factors indicated that he would be at low risk for surgery. The reason for valve replacement was that he was beginning to have symptoms such as shortness of breath and dizziness. Such symptoms indicated that there was obstruction of blood flow through the valve. Left untreated, these symptoms would get worse and he would probably pass out from progressive aortic stenosis, or his condition could develop into congestive heart failure.

In most cases the surgeon just replaces the entire valve by cutting it out of its setting and placing a tissue valve made from biological material (usually from a pig) or with an artificial mechanical valve. The tissue valve can last for 10–15 years. Sometimes, the patient's pulmonary valve is removed and placed in the aortic position, as it will last longer than a pig valve. The pulmonary valve is replaced with another valve from a cadaver. The problem with porcine tissue valves is that they tend to calcify after 10–15 years. They are used usually only in patients who are over 65 years, or in patients who cannot tolerate anticoagulation. The advantage of such tissue valves is that anticoagulation with blood thinners is not required.

Mechanical valves are made from metal and carbon composite materials and are more durable than tissue valves. Mechanical valves are, however, more prone to infection, and there is also a higher tendency to form clots on the valve. Anticoagulants (blood thinners) are needed to prevent clot formation, usually for a lifetime. Otherwise, clots may form, detach, and then lodge in the brain causing a stroke. Blood thinners obviously can cause bleeding if the dose is too high, as the blood can no longer clot as easily. Wounds may not stop bleeding and in some cases spontaneous bleeding into the gut or the brain may cause serious and life-threatening hemorrhages.

Our patient above had two problems with undertaking surgery. He was concerned first about a surgical procedure that has about a 3–5 percent mortality rate, so he sought two additional opinions. Second, he was not sure a pig valve was kosher due to his religious persuasion. Medically, a pig valve was the preferred option because of his advanced age. He was reassured by his rabbi that a porcine valve was not prohibited by his religion. This example demonstrates the complex social and psychological world we live in, how patients make decisions for themselves, and how this also may affect medical decision making by doctors. Some patients may not disclose their real reasons for not following a doctor's guidance in accepting recommendations and may therefore appear to be defiant or to be noncompliant. It is therefore useful for caregivers to take into account nonmedical factors in making recommendations to patients.

It is now also possible to perform mitral and aortic valve procedures using minimally invasive robotic surgery with the da Vinci system. Since this is a relatively new procedure, done only for about 10 years, it is still somewhat experimental in the hands of many surgeons. Complications are related to the experience of the surgeon and that of the institution as a whole.

Congenital Heart Defects

There are several congenital heart defects (CHD) that often cause mixing of oxygen-rich blood with venous or deoxygenated blood due to shunting of blood from the left side of the heart to the right side as described in detail in chapter 7.

Corrective surgical procedures are done as soon as possible after birth if they are serious and incompatible with life. Other procedures are delayed for some years as lesions such as atrial and ventricular septa defects may close with the passage of time. Because of rapid growth in the early years of life, non-life-threatening defects such as aortic coarctation may be corrected when the child grows up as the aorta is expanding and a graft placed early may become too small.

While in many cases operations are needed to correct heart defects, catheter-based procedures are being increasingly utilized. The rationale is that such procedures are easier to perform than surgery because they involve only a needle puncture, which is the catheter's point of insertion. Unlike surgery, catheter-based procedures can also be done repeatedly, if necessary, in a growing child with minimal trauma. This procedure is done by manipulating the tip of the catheter under visual guidance provided by X-rays or echocardiography. Since the chest is not opened to repair the defect, recovery is more rapid. In many pediatric cases of congenital heart disease, catheter and surgical procedures are combined to repair complex heart defects as it is common for a child to have several kinds of defects. The use of catheter-based procedures has become the preferred way to repair less complicated heart defects, such as atrial septal defects.

Details for surgical and catheter treatment of congenital heart disease are covered in greater detail in Chapters 7 and 9. Specific conditions that can be treated with these methods include patent ductus arteriosus, coarctation of the aorta, atrial septal defect, ventricular septal defect, tetralogy of Fallot, and transposition of the great arteries.

Heart Transplants

The first successful organ transplant between a living donor and a patient was a kidney between twins at the Peter Bent Brigham Hospital in Boston in 1954. The transplant was performed by the surgeon Joseph Murray (b. 1919). Murray's partner in this endeavor was the nephrologist John P. Merrill (1917–1984). Murray received a Nobel Prize in 1990 for this accomplishment. After this event, the first organ bank was established in Boston as a result of the growing need for processing organ donation. Organ transplantations involving the liver, heart, lung, pancreas, intestine, and bone marrow have since become widespread.

In situations where cardiomyopathy destroys massive amounts of heart muscle or if there are complex congenital abnormalities, the heart is either replaced via transplantation or an artificial heart is implanted. The first heart transplant was performed by Christiaan Barnard (1922–2001) in South Africa in 1967. He transplanted the heart of a young woman who died in an accident into Louis Washkansky, but Washkansky died from pneumonia 18 days after surgery. The operation was considered a success, as the transplanted heart did not require any external stimulation to support the circulation. This operation also demonstrated that transplantation was a viable idea and survival was indeed feasible. The first heart transplant in the United States was done at the Maimonides Medical Center in New York by Adrian Kantrowitz (1918–2008), on a baby who lived less than seven hours. Now 3,400 heart transplants are done worldwide each year.

Long-term survival is possible after transplantation with the use of immunosuppressive drugs and careful follow-up. Carroll H. Shelby (1923–2012), the famed race car driver, automotive designer, and entrepreneur, had a heart transplant in 1990 and a kidney transplant in 1996. Another well-known American with a heart transplant is John C. Bogle (b. 1929), the founder of the Vanguard Funds, who underwent surgery in 1996 and is alive and doing well at the age of 83. He had right ventricular dysplasia diagnosed in 1982 and experienced half a dozen cardiac arrests due to ventricular fibrillation. Following his transplant in early 1996, he was back at work a month later and was able to play squash three months later. Presently, he still works a full day in the financial industry and admits to feeling more tired than a few years ago, but he is a vigorous 83! Since his transplant he has occasional ventricular premature beats, but no episodes of cardiac arrest have occurred, and he does not have an implantable defibrillator in place.

Though transplantation is the best treatment for severe cardiomyopathy and congestive heart failure, there is a serious limitation of hearts available for transplantation. In the United States alone, there are about 3,000 people on the cardiac waiting list. Since 1990, over 2,000 heart transplants are done annually (2,322 done in 2011), resulting in a shortage of about 1,000 hearts each year. In comparison, about 15,000 kidney transplants have been done annually since 1990.

Patients who qualify for a transplant are placed on a waiting list and notified immediately when a heart is available. The waiting list and donor availability are part of a national allocation system under the guidance of the Organ Procurement and Transplant Network (OPTN). The U.S. Congress created this organization in 1984 to ensure the fair distribution of organs. The United Network for Organ Sharing (UNOS), a nonprofit organization, was awarded the contract by OPTN to manage organ sharing and distribution. UNOS developed an online database system, called UNet, to collect, store, analyze, and publish all OPTN data related to the patient waiting list, organ matching, and transplants. It is a secure, round-the-clock, online information database enabling doctors to register patients for transplants, access all patients already registered for transplants, match organs to waiting patients, and manage critical data before and after their transplants. The United States is divided into 11 regions by UNOS with a total of about 254 transplant centers and 130 heart transplant programs. In each region, there are several independent Organ Procurement Organizations (OPO) based in different cities that inform the UNOS system, so as to organize the delivery of organs when they are available.

There are two main issues facing a patient awaiting a transplant. One is organ shortage and the other is organ rejection if the donor and recipient's immune systems are not compatible. Most adult donor hearts are obtained from healthy accident victims who suffer serious brain injury. Seat belt and helmet laws combined with improved medical care have resulted in fewer deaths, and organs available for transplantation are in short supply. Due to the shortage of organs, a heart may not be available for one to three years.

As there are simply not enough hearts to go around, patients are screened and placed on a scale of priority based on how sick they are. Patients who are listed as 1A are the sickest and are on continuous circulatory support with intravenous medications, have a ventricular assist device, or are on continuous ventilation support with a respirator.

Patients for most kinds of transplants are generally paired by a process called HLA matching. There are protein markers found in most of the body's cells called human leukocyte antigen (HLA). Such markers are important when matching patients and donors for bone marrow, peripheral blood cell transfusions, cord blood, and bone marrow transplant. A transplant center examines how similar the HLA tissue types of the patient and the donor are. Long-term success of a transplant depends on a high degree of compatibility between the donor's organ and the patient's immune system. Otherwise there is a good chance that the organ will be rejected. However, for heart patients HLA testing is often not needed. Instead a panel reactive antibody (PRA) blood test is done for screening. The PRA test is given as a score from 0 to 99 percent and more detailed tests may be needed if the score is over 25 percent. If the PRA score is over 50 percent, transplantation may not be done as there is a high probability of rejection of the heart.

When a donor heart becomes available, the surgeons or their assistants research the data on the UNOS computer system and find a suitable recipient. Ideally, donor hearts have to be free of heart disease, be matched for size, be less than 65 years of age, and must not have experienced loss of circulation for more than four hours. The donor has to qualify for brain death, though he or she may still be on mechanical ventilation. The donor has to be free of hepatitis and HIV/AIDS.

The recipient's hospital team then travels to the intended donor's hospital and ascertains that the patient has been legally declared brain dead. They then inject the heart with potassium chloride to arrest it, remove the heart from the chest, pack it in a cold container, and transport it back to their own hospital by ambulance or private aircraft. The heart needs to be implanted within four to six hours after being removed from the donor. The remaining organs may be distributed to patients at other sites in a similar manner.

Each potential recipient candidate has already been physically and psychologically screened and briefed extensively about the surgery and what to expect. They should be nonalcoholic, ideally drug-free, and healthy in other respects. The intended recipient carries communication equipment so he or she can be contacted immediately by the hospital, enabling prompt arrival and preparation for transplant surgery. Psychological support is provided by the nurse coordinator as surgery has to be done very quickly with little warning and patients can become emotionally fragile in this situation.

After induction of anesthesia, the entire heart and the great vessels are excised with the patient on cardiopulmonary bypass. The back of the left atrium with the four pulmonary veins are left in place and the donor heart attached to the great vessels of the recipient and to the remaining part of the left atrium. This procedure is called *orthotopic transplantation*. In some cases, the failing heart is left in place and the transplanted heart attached to the great vessels so that there is a double heart. This procedure is referred to as *heterotropic transplantation* as the patient's heart is not removed. If the donor heart is rejected, it is removed and the patient still has his or her own heart. The patient's own heart also has a chance to recover and become functional over time, as it may in some cases.

The donor heart is warmed and restarted, electrically if necessary, and the patient taken off the bypass machine once the heart starts beating. The patient recovers in the cardiac intensive care unit and is discharged in 10 to 14 days if there are no complications. The patient has already been started on immunosuppressive drugs to prevent rejection and these are continued. Frequent checks are made for signs of rejection, and the heart muscle is regularly biopsied for microscopic signs of rejection. A cardiac rehabilitation program is very important to get the patient back to a regular exercise routine. The cost of a heart transplant in the United States including surgery, medications, tests, and follow-up visits for the first year is approximately $1 million.

Pericardial Disease

The pericardium is a thin transparent membrane surrounding the heart, and it is not an essential structure for normal functioning of the heart. There are two layers (outer and inner) and there is a small amount of fluid between these two layers. The pericardium may become inflamed due to viral or tuberculosis infections, cancer deposits, or unknown causes. The amount of fluid between the two layers increases during inflammation and produces a *pericardial effusion*. Given that the pericardium is essentially a tight sac, the fluid causes compression of the heart by preventing expansion of the ventricles during systole. The fluid accumulation interferes with the heart's ability to pump blood properly due to cardiac compression. If left untreated, the reduction in cardiac output leads to low blood pressure that can be dangerous and cause death.

Pericardial effusion is usually treated by the insertion of a needle under the front of the rib cage to drain the excess fluid. The procedure is called *pericardiocentesis*. Sometimes, the fluid reaccumulates after removal and the condition becomes repetitive and chronic. In such cases, a procedure called a *pericardial window* is done to relieve cardiac compression. In this procedure, the surgeon makes an incision under the rib cage and cuts away a portion of the pericardium to create a more permanent opening for drainage of fluid into the space surrounding the heart. This procedure allows any fluid to escape into the lung cavity, avoiding accumulation of fluid around the heart and preventing the heart from being compressed.

A pericardial window is also done in cases when the pericardium is calcified. This condition is called *constrictive pericarditis*. A cause for calcification of the pericardium may not be found, but it most likely occurs after undetected viral infections. In these cases, the hardening of the pericardial sac also leads to a reduction in the pumping action of the heart. Since this problem leads to low blood pressure, the pericardium needs to be cut into and stripped off the heart to allow it to pump normally.

Performing a pericardial window requires a fairly large incision and a certain period of recovery. With minimally invasive robotic surgery (e.g., the da Vinci Surgical System), the procedure is less invasive and recovery is much more rapid due to a smaller incision. The patient recovers more quickly, can be discharged the next day and is able to return to normal activity and work much earlier than with open chest surgery.

POSTOPERATIVE RECOVERY PERIOD

Postoperative care is crucial in ensuring successful recovery from surgery. With modern anesthesia, careful surgical technique, and close intraoperative monitoring, surgery today is actually incredibly safe 95–99 percent of the time (in nonemergency cases). Many of the outcomes and successes of modern surgery are actually due to improvements in our understanding of what can go wrong during the postoperative phase, such as wound infections, pneumonia, pulmonary embolism, and bleeding. This phase of surgical care is often almost exclusively in the hands of highly skilled, specially trained nurses and physical therapists.

Following surgery, the patient is transferred to the Post-Anesthesia Care Unit (PACU) or directly to the Cardiothoracic Intensive Care (CTIC) Unit. After observation for 12–24 hours to ensure that the anesthesia wears off and that the patient's vital signs are stable, the endotracheal tube is removed to allow the patient to breathe spontaneously. Supplemental oxygen is delivered via a face mask. Blood pressure, heart rate, temperature, oxygen saturation, and carbon dioxide blood levels are continuously monitored to make sure that these parameters are in the normal range. Abnormalities in these indices may be a warning that there is a problem with congestive heart failure, a collapsed lung, or an infection. Oral and intravenous fluid intake, drainage from the chest wound, and urinary output are also monitored so that the intake and output of fluids are carefully balanced. A bedside computer tracks all of these variables in a sequential manner so that caregivers can review how the patient has been progressing as the hours and days pass.

If minimally invasive or "keyhole" surgery was done, the patient can be discharged as early as the next day. For open-heart surgery, the patient is kept in hospital for about four to five days postoperatively to ensure there is no fever, bleeding, heart failure, or heart rhythm disturbance. The chest drainage tubes and the pacemaker wires are removed when they are no longer needed. Feeding is commenced only when the patient is fully awake, able to breathe and swallow on his own, and is no longer nauseous. Oral fluids and soft pureed foods are followed by solid food when the patient can tolerate a more regular diet.

Medications are often needed for pain control and, sometimes, for congestive heart failure or heart rhythm abnormalities that occur postoperatively. Physical therapy to get the patient moving is commenced, often only a couple of days after surgery. Movement reduces complications such as pneumonia and clot formation (*thrombophlebitis*) in the leg and pelvic veins. Clots from the legs and pelvis may detach and travel to the lungs and cause death from pulmonary embolism. In many cases following uncomplicated heart surgery, the patient is out of bed the day following surgery, and home in 3–5 days. It is remarkable how strong and resilient the heart really is, and how quickly it can recover from major surgery and allow the owner to get back to early physical activity.

Upon discharge, the patient is given guidelines for physical and sexual activity, diet, how to take medications, and when to call for help. The patient is also briefed on wound care and possible situations that will require immediate attention, along with instructions on how to get medical help if necessary. The patient will be seen by the surgeon and the cardiologist about a month after discharge for a postoperative check if there are no complications. The cardiologist is primarily responsible for long-term follow-up and ongoing care.

Cardiac rehabilitation as an outpatient is strongly recommended when full healing has occurred to speed up recovery and reduce recurrence of coronary artery disease. It is important to provide teaching about risk factor reduction in terms of diet, exercise, and abstaining from tobacco, and to emphasize that early recurrence will occur if these guidelines are not followed closely.

COMPLICATIONS OF CARDIAC SURGERY

Any surgical intervention on the human body can result in complications. Though most patients would take any complication as being serious, from a medical standpoint, complications after surgery are classified as being either non-life-threatening complications and life-threatening. However, some non-life-threatening complications can become serious if left untreated.

Non-Life-Threatening Complications

Non-life-threatening complications are often self-limited and clear up with time or with treatment. Common non-life-threatening complications are listed as follows:

- Minor wound infection
- Bleeding from the surgical sites
- Bruising
- Allergies to tape and medications
- Minor blood transfusion reactions
- Atrial fibrillation and other atrial arrhythmias
- Pneumonia
- Temporary confusion and psychosis
- Alcohol withdrawal symptoms

Occasionally, the patient may develop fever and pericarditis with chest pain, known as *post-pericardiotomy syndrome*. This condition is due to inflammation of the pericardium and the pleural covering of the lungs. Though the exact cause is not known, it is believed that antibodies to the heart develop as a result of surgical injury and an autoimmune condition results. Usually, the condition resolves in three weeks or so. If a lot of fluid accumulates around the heart and lungs, it is removed with a needle or a pericardial window is created surgically.

Other complications include depression, impotence in men, and insomnia for weeks or months after surgery. If depression and/or impotence are serious, the person needs to be referred to a specialist to help treat the condition. Depression may require treatment with medications as it is linked to increased risk of death in patients with heart disease. Most of these complications are treated in the immediate postoperative period without long-lasting complications. Some treatments will need to be continued as an outpatient with appropriate consultations.

Major and Life-Threatening Complications

Life-threatening complications include cardiac arrest, rupture of sutures, dehiscence of valves or grafts or major bleeding, all of which can cause death. Major complications may result in delayed recovery, debilitation due to permanent damage to the brain or other organs, or in death. The death rate for coronary artery bypass surgery is 2–3 percent. Death rates are lower than this rate if the patient is healthy and young. The death rate is higher in older patients, if the general health of the patient is poor, when left ventricular function is seriously impaired, or if the surgery is complicated and prolonged.

It is important to realize that over a period of 10 years, the mortality rate is approximately the same for medically and surgically treated patients, at about 3.3–3.4 percent per year. In this context, in the case of a patient with serious heart disease, the risk of surgery is often worthwhile if the patient's quality of life can be improved. This is especially true if the patient is younger, physically active, or travels a great deal, so that taking medications several times a day becomes tedious and difficult to maintain.

Some surgical procedures, such as the correction of congenital heart disease, can damage the electrical system of the heart. This results in a condition called "heart block," where not all the impulses from the sinoatrial node get through to the heart to make it pump at a normal rate. This condition will require correction with implantation of a temporary or permanent pacemaker.

One of the most serious complications of heart surgery is stroke, often with a corresponding cognitive impairment involving a loss of memory and an inability to function intellectually. This situation results from atheroma that line aorta and other large blood vessels with popcorn-like deposits of cholesterol. These deposits flake off when the vessels are manipulated, or when catheters and tubes are passed through them during surgery. The flakes that break off travel to the brain, obstruct the cerebral circulation, and cause strokes. This complication happens in about 2–3 percent of patients undergoing cardiac surgery of all types.

Another problem arises from the clotting of blood platelets, which occurs as a result of being on a bypass machine. These are actually mini-clots that lodge in the blood vessels in the brain and cause neurological damage. Low blood pressure during surgery aggravates this condition due to sluggish blood flow through the brain, causing reduced perfusion with oxygen.

This condition, colloquially known as *pump head*, results in cognitive impairment and occurs in as many as 30 percent of patients in some cases. Patients may show confusion, memory loss, insomnia, serious mood changes, depression, lack of impulse control, socially and sexually inappropriate behavior, and outbursts of rage and anger. These emotional side effects may occur immediately after surgery, or become more apparent only months later, which can result in long-term permanent disability. There is no cure for this condition and the symptoms may actually get worse with time. These complications need to be prevented at the time of surgery with careful attention to adequate technique intraoperatively involving adequate anticoagulation, maintaining adequate oxygenation, blood pressure, and perfusion with the bypass pump. Psychiatric and psychological consultation, support, and medications are useful in managing depression and mood changes.

Postoperatively, one of the most serious complications is thrombophlebitis or clot formation in the leg and pelvic veins. If these clots detach and are carried to the lungs, they cause a condition known as *pulmonary embolism*. When pulmonary embolism is massive, it can cause death due to blockage of the pulmonary artery, blocking outflow of blood from the right ventricle to the lungs. If the condition is less severe, it is treated with heparin and other blood thinners. In cases of massive emoblization to the pulmonary arteries, surgical removal of the clot is required. Early mobilization after surgery is key to preventing clotting in the leg and pelvic veins.

With careful preoperative assessment, intraoperative monitoring, and postoperative care, it is possible to reduce both minor and major complications. Complications can be anticipated and prevented, or early intervention and treatment can avoid catastrophic outcomes.

SUMMARY

In a little over 150 years, the development of anesthesia, antisepsis, and blood transfusion has transformed surgical approaches to disease dramatically. However, it is only in the lifetime of most living physicians that modern cardiac surgery has become routine because of advances in modern technology.

Surgical treatment of heart disease has seen tremendous strides, especially in the past 75 years, and millions of people all over the world have had congenital heart defects fixed, coronary artery disease corrected with bypass grafts, and valvular disease repaired. Cardiac transplants have dramatically saved patients who would otherwise have died. Surgery, in most of these cases, has not only corrected the underlying problems, but has prolonged and improved the quality of life. One major factor is cost: cardiac testing and treatments are very expensive. However, the economic dividend of treating people in their most productive years of working life must also be considered as this offsets the costs of treatment.

11

Cardiac Arrest and Resuscitation

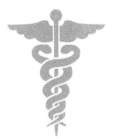

Calvin was 21 when he collapsed on the soccer field. Fortunately, it was near the college campus, where he was an engineering student. Another student had the sense to call 911, though she did not know what had happened. The city emergency medical team arrived within minutes. Bystander cardiopulmonary resuscitation (CPR) was started on the scene, and within 10 minutes an advanced cardiac life support (ACLS) ambulance arrived. The cardiac monitor showed ventricular fibrillation. The emergency medical technician defibrillated the heart with 360 joules of current and Calvin was immediately revived. After being admitted to hospital, he was evaluated by a cardiologist. The electrocardiogram showed no abnormality. Cardiac enzymes were normal. so no heart damage had occurred. Calvin had a 24-hour Holter monitor strapped on in the hospital and no important abnormality was found. He did not undergo an exercise stress test during that admission to hospital. An echocardiogram was completely normal, so he was discharged with no medications.

I saw Calvin three months after this episode and found him to be a tall, fit-looking young man, with an easy, quiet, and thoughtful manner. He could not remember much about the cardiac arrest. The week before the incident he had been studying late for finals, had felt exhausted, and was sleep deprived. However, he was doing very well in school and expected to graduate the following year. There were absolutely no abnormal physical findings. His blood pressure and heart examination were completely normal. However, he admitted to using LSD on and off. On the night before the soccer game he had a several "hits" of LSD, as he called it, and briefly passed out for a while. He also admitted to using cocaine occasionally. After the cardiac arrest, he stopped all drug use.

The EKG, exercise stress test, Holter monitor, and two-dimensional echocardiogram were all within normal limits. These tests essentially showed he had no structural heart disorder. Was this a one-time event or something that could recur and cause death if unattended?

I discussed with Calvin the various reasons why fibrillation may occur in an otherwise healthy person. This arrhythmia does occur during drug use and, in fact, is often the cause of death in drug overdose. Though it was by no means certain, I thought that his heart may have been damaged by drug use, I advised electrophysiologic testing and this test may or may not indicate he needed an implantable defibrillator. However, he did not think that he wanted to have testing done and declined this option. On follow-up for two years, he remained healthy.

The heart is unique among organs in that it directly sustains life, and the cessation of its action leads to death rapidly. Paradoxically, however, it also has the ability to electrocute itself and kill its owner very quickly. The rhythm disorder that most often causes self-electrocution is ventricular fibrillation (VF), a chaotically disruptive rhythm that will lead to death 99.9 percent of the time unless it is terminated. The heart undergoes very rapid uncoordinated electrical activity in VF, so that there is no effective pumping activity to eject blood. The end result is rapid loss of consciousness and death. If the heart stops for more than a few minutes, there is irreversible brain damage due to lack of oxygen.

Ventricular fibrillation is the most common rhythm responsible for *sudden cardiac death* (SCD), when someone drops dead. If Calvin had not been revived immediately by CPR and defibrillation, he would certainly be dead today. In the United States, out of a population of just over 300 million, it is estimated that about 240,000 cardiac arrests were treated in 2005. In 2011, the number was probably closer to 300,000 cases of cardiac arrest. In Europe, it is estimated that there were about 450,000 cardiac arrests out of a population of 455 million in 2005. At present, over three-quarters of a million people die suddenly from cardiac arrest in the Western world each year.

What is remarkable about SCD is that there are often no symptoms before cardiac arrest occurs. Up to 80 percent of people who die from cardiac arrest have coronary artery disease as the underlying cause. However, two-thirds of those who are resuscitated do not have acute myocardial infarction, as was the case with Calvin. Hypertrophic cardiomyopathy, mitral valve prolapse, and other valve diseases account for about 5 percent each in causing SCD. In about 5 percent, the cause of cardiac arrest is unknown and the heart seems anatomically normal. The age range in adults is about 45 to 75 years of age. Among the young, SCD accounts for a fifth of deaths from age 1 to 13 years, and 30 percent from ages 14 to 21 years of age.

SCD leads to more deaths than any other cause in both the United States and Europe. It is a catastrophic and shocking occurrence since the person seems perfectly healthy and then, within minutes, is gone forever. Since the peak age of sudden death is around the age of 55, these people are not really old or elderly. Given that SCD strikes men and women in the prime of life, and in their most productive years, these deaths represent a significant toll both socially and economically. A lot of effort has, therefore, gone into reaching cardiac arrest victims quickly to treat them when cardiac arrest occurs.

The majority of cardiac arrests arise from disorders in electrical activity within the ventricles of the heart. Rarely, the problem starts in the atria (e.g., when the person has a condition such as Wolff-Parkinson-White syndrome as described in Chapter 6). Unless proven otherwise, when someone "drops dead" it is presumed that death was due to very rapid ventricular tachycardia (VT) that degenerated into VF, or that the heart developed VF directly (Figure 11.1).

These two abnormal rhythms, VT and VF, can be shocked back into a normal rhythm with a defibrillator. In a minority of cases, the heart stops completely with no electrical action at all. The absence of any rhythm is called *asystole*, and the EKG shows a *flat line*. Asystole cannot be shocked into a normal rhythm with a defibrillator, as the heart is basically electrically and mechanically inactive. In a minority of cases of asystole, a pacemaker may restore cardiac activity, but only if the stoppage is due to conduction system disease and not if the heart has lost all of its intrinsic electrical activity. This situation occurs as a terminal event when the heart is heavily damaged and there is a massive loss of heart muscle tissue.

The evolution of the use of electricity to restore cardiac activity in VF and VT is one of the most fascinating stories in medicine. It involves the discovery of electricity, the long road to discovering how electricity causes VF, and how, oddly enough, electricity itself can be used to shock the heart back to life. These discoveries occurred over hundreds of years and have the characteristics of a near-miracle, as it is literally a form of reanimation that brings a person back to life.

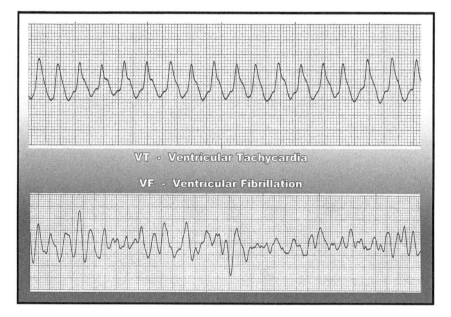

Figure 11.1 Upper panel: Regular ventricular tachycardia at 180 beats per minute. Lower panel: Ventricular fibrillation. © Steve Allen/Dreamstime.com.

EARLY HISTORY OF RESUSCITATION

The fact that VF can be reversed using electricity is one the great triumphs of the scientific method, modern medicine, and biomedical engineering. The discovery that the heart is an electromechanical pump, and that external electrical currents can be used to reverse VF, is a remarkable story with many actors.

We should go back 2,500 years to the ancient Greeks who knew that rubbing certain materials together such as amber could cause an electric charge to occur. Electrical sparking happens quite suddenly if two such objects are brought close together. William Gilbert, the Royal Physician to Queen Elizabeth I, had studied the electrical properties of amber and the magnetic properties of the lodestone in the 16th century. He thought of the earth as a gigantic magnet with two poles at each end. He coined the term *electricity* and also introduced the terms *electric force*, *electrical attraction*, and *magnetic pole*. The great English scientist Michael Faraday (1791–1867) correlated the relationship between magnetism and electricity. Though he had no formal education, he discovered *electromagnetic induction* and was the first to invent the electric motor, the generator, and the transformer. These discoveries opened the way for the electrification of homes, factories, and transportation, and led to the invention of several electrical tools, machines, and devices in the 19th and 20th centuries.

The Leyden jar, invented in 1745, was the first device able to store and discharge electricity, and it was able to deliver a considerable electric shock. Basically, it was a primitive capacitor that could accumulate and store electricity when charged by an electrostatic generator that worked through friction and generated electricity by mechanical rotations. The jar was mostly a curiosity and used for amusement to shock people and animals at social events, such as at parties at the French court. Benjamin Franklin, who was present at the royal court and famously experimented with electricity during thunderstorms, linked a group of Leyden jars in series and called it a *battery*. A less fortunate fellow experimenter, the German-Russian Georg Wilhelm Richmann, was killed by lightning in 1753 while experimenting during a thunderstorm in St. Petersburg. His clothes were burned, his skin singed, and his shoes blown apart. He was basically fried by the electric thunderbolt.

In 1788, Charles Kite reported in the *Register of the Royal Humane Society of London* that a child who fell out of a window was allegedly revived by the application of electrical shocks. His account contains a diagram of an electrical device showing a Leyden jar with attached electrodes that could have functioned as a primitive defibrillator. A certain Mr. Squires was credited with the remarkable feat of reviving the child. He applied shocks using the jar to various parts of the body. They failed to have any effect until the shocks were applied to the chest. A pulse was detected and the child recovered after being unconscious for a full 20 minutes. Though this event is often quoted as the "first successful" human resuscitation, it is highly unlikely a true case of revival by the use of electricity. The delay involved was too long and the child would have been dead or severely brain damaged if cardiac arrest had occurred. It is more likely that the child was dazed by a concussion and recovered spontaneously.

In the mid-1700s, a series of humane societies sprang up in European capitals with the goal of reviving those who had drowned. Initially, mouth-to-mouth respiration was recommended. However, in 1782, the Royal Humane Society of London changed its preference to manual assistance using an air bellows. Despite this, any bystander could still use the mouth-to-mouth breathing method. Though it is unlikely that assisted respiration alone would have any significant effect in reversing cardiac arrest, it was recognized that proper ventilation was an essential part of resuscitation.

The awareness that electricity caused death probably led to the idea that electricity itself could be used to shock the victim back to life again. In 1775 a veterinarian and physician, Peter Christian Abildgaard (1740–1801) in Denmark, did the first real experiments on the effects of electric shock on animals. He found that he could render chickens senseless with an electrical shock. Upon applying another shock, the apparently lifeless chickens were sometimes revived. Those that recovered seemed healthy and one even went on to lay an egg. Abildgaard made two other key observations. While the hens could be rendered senseless by a shock to the head, a shock to the thorax was needed to revive them. Second, when he shocked hens and left them overnight, he found they were completely dead and not revivable with shocks the next morning. However, when he delivered a second shock several minutes after the first, revival was successful. The conclusion was that the first shock produced a state that was reversible by a second shock for only a short time. After this window of opportunity was lost, the bird was permanently dead.

Abildgaard made some other astute conclusions from his experiments. He knew that death from lightning often left no trace in the body upon dissection. Therefore, whatever effect electrical shocks had on the body, it was something that was similar to what lightning did when it struck a person. He also surmised correctly that such a condition could be reversed with electrical shocks, as he had demonstrated, but only if it was done quickly. It was also logical to assume that the heart was involved in death from electrical shock, as only shocks to the chest were effective in reviving his chickens. Early experimenters did not know that death was due to VF provoked by electricity, as Carl Ludwig in Leipzig only discovered this arrhythmia in 1849.

EVOLUTION OF DEFIBRILLATION IN THE 20TH CENTURY

It took several different researchers to bring defibrillation to a practical clinical reality. In 1889, Jean-Louis Prevost (who trained with the French neurophysiologist Alfred Vulpian) and Frederic Battelli, two physicians in Geneva, showed low electrical currents provoked VF and high electrical currents terminated it. This was a key discovery that led to the development of the defibrillator by other workers. The work of Prevost and Battelli influenced a Russian junior colleague, Lina S. Schtern (1878-1968). After returning to Moscow, she tasked her graduate student Naum Gurvich (1905–1981) to continue research on the effects of electricity on dogs, sheep, and goats. Gurvich and his colleague G. S. Yuniev showed that shocks of 2,000–6,000 volts from a direct current (DC) capacitor were superior to alternating current (AC) capacitors in terminating VF. Later, Gurvich added an inductance coil to the circuit to dampen and smooth out the high-voltage spike produced by the capacitor alone and prolong it by milliseconds. The addition of the inductance coil reduced heart damage caused by the high-voltage spike. This innovation essentially created the Gurvich biphasic waveform that is still used today in most external defibrillators. By 1952, his DC defibrillator was in wide clinical use in the Soviet Union.

In the late 1950s, Bohumil Peleška, a Czech physician who visited Gurvich in Moscow, also experimented with adding an inductance coil to the DC circuit. He essentially confirmed that this addition optimized the discharge and reduced cardiac damage by allowing the use of lower voltages. He also showed that the heart was more likely to go back into VF if the shock was delivered in the recovery phase. This is the where the *vulnerable period* of the ventricle occurs, as described later.

The focus turned to humans in the 1880s during the electrification of railways, factories, and homes. The Consolidated Electric Company of New York and the Edison Company of New York became concerned because linemen were dropping dead when accidentally electrocuted. The company approached William Bennett Kouwenhoven (1886–1975) at Johns Hopkins University in Baltimore to help with this problem. He and his colleagues, D.R. Hooker, G. Knickerbocker, and O.R. Langworthy, designed an AC defibrillator that worked on animals to terminate VF.

They also discovered the basic elements of external cardiopulmonary resuscitation (CPR) by chest compression quite by serendipity in 1960. During experiments on defibrillation, Guy Knickerbocker noted something interesting while placing electrodes on the chest of animals to deliver an electrical shock. In this experiment, blood pressure was measured by a gauge connected to a catheter in the femoral artery. The blood pressure gauge registered a blip when the electrode was applied to the chest and pressed down with some force. A pulse was also detectable in the femoral artery in the groin. They realized that firm chest compression with their hands had the same effect. Thus, external cardiopulmonary resuscitation (CPR) was born. Basically, the heart is squeezed between the sternum and the spine when force is applied to the sternum by pumping the chest. Bystanders are now taught to do chest compressions to maintain circulation during cardiac arrest until advanced life support, including defibrillation, becomes available.

In 1947, Claude Beck (1894–1971), a surgeon in Cleveland, Ohio, defibrillated the first human heart during open-heart surgery. He was operating on a 17-year-old male and cardiac arrest occurred while he was closing the chest. He reopened the chest and, using a defibrillator he had devised, defibrillated the heart successfully. The patient survived and lived for many years to become the first authentic case of human cardiac resuscitation from VF.

In 1956, Paul Zoll (1911–1999), at the Beth Israel Hospital and Harvard Medical School in Boston, also constructed an AC defibrillator. He was the first to defibrillate a human heart externally through the intact chest in 1956. However, AC defibrillation was unreliable as it did not always succeed in terminating VF. The use of AC sometimes leads to the heart going back into VF as the electrical pulse is too long and causes refibrillation, as Gurvich and Peleška had already found. Today, all defibrillators use direct current.

The idea that atrial tachycardias and stable VT could be stopped electively by electricity was a novel concept at that time. In 1959, A. A. Vishnevskii, B. M. Tsukerman, and S. M. Smelovskii in the Soviet Union reported in the Russian literature that atrial fibrillation could be terminated with DC shock. Until about 1960, electricity was used to terminate arrhythmias only on an emergency basis in the United States. Bernard Lown (b. 1921) and his colleagues Sidney Alexander and Robert Kleiger were the first to electively terminate VT by using an AC defibrillator in 1960, at the Peter Bent Brigham Hospital in Boston. The patient remained in persistent VT despite large doses of procainamide. In a bold and daring move, Lown took sole responsibility for administering electric shock that successfully terminated VT without any dire consequences and with full recovery of the patient. This was a remarkable achievement given that VT is a very serious arrhythmia that often leads to death if left untreated.

Barouh Berkovits (b. 1926), a Czech-American engineer working in Buffalo, New York, who was aware of Gurvich's and Peleška's work, constructed a DC defibrillator based on the same electrical circuit using a capacitor and an inductance coil that delivered a damped half-sinusoidal waveform. This device was later tested by Bernard Lown at the Peter Bent Brigham Hospital and the Harvard School of Public Health in Boston. After extensive testing, they introduced DC defibrillators in the United States, as they were safer and more effective than AC devices.

After the successful termination of VT using an AC defibrillator, Lown conceived the idea of delivering a single electrical pulse from a DC device to terminate arrhythmias other than VF. He introduced a timing device that delayed discharge of the shock to coincide with the R-wave of the EKG to avoid striking the T-wave during the *vulnerable period*. The characteristics of the *vulnerable period* are described later in this chapter. This innovation, named *cardioversion* by Lown, made termination of arrhythmias such as atrial tachycardia, atrial fibrillation, and VT both practical and safe. Today, all advanced life-support ambulances, critical care units, and some public areas, such as airports and stadiums, have cardioverter-defibrillators available for the immediate treatment of people suffering from cardiac arrhythmias.

ELECTROPHYSIOLOGY OF CARDIAC ARREST

Ventricular fibrillation is a chaotic, uncoordinated action of the heart so that the heart looks like "a bag of worms." Back in 1889, even before the EKG was invented, John MacWilliam (1857–1937), a Scottish physiologist and physician, had already surmised that sudden death in humans was caused by VF. Some 70 years later, in the 1960s, after the EKG and the defibrillator were available to record and treat VF, he was proved right. By then, out-of-hospital resuscitation programs in Seattle, Minneapolis, and Belfast were started in the 1960s and 1970s to revive victims of cardiac arrest. It was only then that VF was found to be the commonest cause of death during cardiac arrest.

This rhythm disturbance causes the heart to quiver fruitlessly 500–600 times a minute in a completely disorganized manner so that blood cannot be pumped out of the heart. This rhythm was only a laboratory curiosity when it was first discovered. Carl Ludwig (1816–1895) and Mauritius Hoffa in Leipzig exposed this arrhythmia in 1849, when they found they could reliably cause VF by applying an electrical stimulus directly to the heart. For some time this arrhythmia had a variety of different names. In 1874, Alfred Vulpian (1826–1887) christened this arrhythmia *mouvement fibrillaire* ("fibrillary movement"). Today. we use a modification of the French name and call this rhythm *ventricular fibrillation*.

The brilliant young physiologist George Ralph Mines (1886–1914) made a key discovery on the genesis of VF in 1913 while working at a marine research laboratory in Roscoff, Brittany. For several years at the University of Cambridge, England, he had been working on frog, electric ray, and rabbit hearts. He showed that VF occurred only when an external electrical stimulus fell on the T-wave of the electrocardiogram. He discovered that there is a small window called the *vulnerable period* just before the apex of the T-wave, when the heart muscle is recovering, and just after it has depolarized electrically to cause ventricular contraction. Mines showed by his experimental work that if an external electrical stimulus were delivered to the heart during this narrow vulnerable period, VF was triggered and death of the animal would occur. Even today, this discovery remains one of the great cornerstones of cardiac electrophysiology.

The problem with AC defibrillators was that the electrical pulse would provoke VF soon after terminating it initially. The reason was that the continuous sinusoidal AC pulse was so long that it would traverse the vulnerable periods of normal beats that followed after VF was successfully terminated, thereby throwing the heart back into fibrillation. This problem did not occur with DC defibrillators as a single short pulse was delivered. Knowledge of the existence of the vulnerable period led to the modification of the DC defibrillator by Bernard Lown by including a timing delay switch to allow discharge to occur on the R-wave. This innovation allowed for the safe discharge of the device to stop arrhythmias by avoiding the vulnerable period.

Tragically, Mines died very shortly following this discovery at the age of 28, when he was found unconscious in his laboratory at McGill University in

Montreal. Apparently, he was experimenting on himself when he died, as he was found with an intravenous line he had presumably placed himself in one of his veins. Unfortunately, he never lived to know that he had made one of the greatest discoveries in cardiac electrophysiology.

Cardiac arrest from VF can occur spontaneously when the myocardium becomes unstable due to cardiac damage during myocardial ischemia or infarction, and in cardiomyopathy. The heart is unable to maintain electrical integrity and the normal electrical process of depolarization and repolarization is disrupted, so that it becomes electrically unstable. This condition leads to spontaneous VF.

Cardiac arrest can also be caused by ventricular premature beats. Sometimes the heart misfires and an extra beat—a ventricular premature beat—may spontaneously erupt from the ventricles during the *vulnerable period*. Such premature beats trigger VT that often degenerates into VF. In this way, the heart basically electrocutes itself.

There are two varieties of VT: regular and irregular. During VT, the heart may beat regularly but rapidly, from rates between 100 beats per minute to 300 or more per minute (see Figure 11.1, upper panel). When the rate is slower and regular, the patient does not lose consciousness and CPR is not needed. In such cases, intravenous and oral medications such as amiodarone, sotalol, and procainamide can be used to terminate and control the arrhythmia. If medications are not effective, electrical treatment with cardioversion is performed. Permanent abolition of the arrhythmia can be obtained by radiofrequency ablation by destroying the electrical pathway that allows the circular rotation of the rhythm through the electrical conduction system in the ventricles.

The second variety of VT is rapid and irregular, causing the patient to lose consciousness if it continues for a minute or more. This variety of VT can degenerate quickly into VF. This condition is called *pulseless* VT when it is sustained and the patient passes out. In rapid pulseless VT, the abnormal rhythm is treated immediately by external defibrillation in the same manner as VF. An implantable defibrillator may be needed to prevent future cardiac arrest.

Today it is known that approximately 25 percent of people who die from CAD just drop dead with no prior symptoms whatsoever. The only practical way to revive them is by defibrillation. After revival, patients are studied in the catheterization and electrophysiology laboratory. These tests will help uncover underlying disease conditions and help to guide the choice of treatment.

CAUSES OF SUDDEN CARDIAC DEATH

Coronary Artery Disease

Sudden death from VF occurs most often because of underlying coronary heart disease. As noted earlier, in two-thirds of people with cardiac arrest, there is no heart damage (i.e., a myocardial infarction, commonly referred to as a *heart attack*) when they are resuscitated, though they have coronary disease. In the remaining third of the patients, VF occurs mostly during the early phase of a myocardial infarction.

In those people who do not evolve a myocardial infarction after they are resuscitated, there may have been sudden slight disruptions of blood flow leading to ischemia, not enough to cause infarction, but enough to lead to electrical instability and VF. It is also possible that there are transient risk factors that destabilize myocardium that is already electrically unstable. Such risk factors may include psychological stress or other states that increase cardiac sympathetic nervous system discharge and high levels of adrenaline that provoke VF. There may also be other transient risk factors that remain to be identified.

Cardiomyopathy

Ventricular fibrillation can result from cardiomyopathy as damage to heart muscle causes electrical instability, and this condition is a necessary precursor to VF. Heart muscle damage results from conditions such as myocarditis, due to infections or cardiomyopathy. Alcohol is a common cause of cardiomyopathy as alcohol depresses heart muscle function and also damages it, even if the person is not an alcoholic. Viruses and Chagas disease (due to a trypanosome parasite) can cause serious heart muscle disease. Some anticancer drugs, such as adriamycin and cyclophosphamide, damage the heart. Certain toxic chemicals and heavy metals, such as carbon tetrachloride and cobalt, can also cause heart muscle damage. Peripartum cardiomyopathy occurs in women in the last month of pregnancy, or in the five months after childbirth, and cardiac arrest has been reported in some such cases. Postpartum cardiomyopathy often resolves spontaneously several months after delivery.

A common feature in cardiomyopathy is congestive heart failure that may be severe if the heart is badly damaged. In some cases cardiomyopathy is reversible and if VF occurs a decision needs to be made if a defibrillator should be implanted.

Genetic Electrical Abnormalities

Genetic abnormalities, such as the long QT interval syndrome and Brugada syndrome, are due to genetic or chromosome aberration, and can cause sudden death in children and young adults. Over a dozen genetic abnormalities cause prolongation of the ventricular action potential resulting in the long QT-interval syndrome (LQTS). Jervell-Lange-Nielsen syndrome is an autosomal recessive form of LQTS associated with congenital deafness. Romano-Ward syndrome is an autosomal dominant form that is not associated with deafness. In LQTS there is a marked propensity for ventricular arrhythmias and half the afflicted children die before reaching adulthood. Exercise and surges in adrenaline due to acute psychological stress can provoke VT or VF in vulnerable hearts and cause sudden loss of consciousness or cardiac arrest.

Brugada syndrome is another inherited genetic abnormality that causes sudden death, chiefly affecting young men. There are characteristic changes in the EKG showing elevation of the ST-segments in certain leads. As with LQTS, genetic testing can be done to confirm the diagnosis.

Idiopathic Causes

Idiopathic VF refers to cardiac arrest occurring when no definite cause can be identified. This condition occurs in about 1 percent of cases of cardiac arrest. The heart is "normal" as far as cardiac testing can disclose, but something that is not identifiable must be present. In our case above, Calvin may have had idiopathic VF, or it could be related to drug abuse that caused microscopic damage to his heart. In some cases, certain genetic abnormalities and the long QT interval syndrome have been uncovered as the cause of cardiac arrest or death, and in such cases, in what was once classified as idiopathic, a biological cause was identified. It is likely that with further research, causes will be found in "idiopathic" VF in the future.

Drugs and Chemicals

A number of drugs used for treatment of various medical conditions can also cause VF. Diuretics used for treating hypertension and congestive heart failure sometimes lead to a low blood potassium. Low blood potassium levels predispose to cell membrane electrical instability and lead to cardiac arrest. Potassium replacement during diuretic therapy is crucial to preventing cardiac arrest. Psychotropic drugs, such as trifluoperazine and trazodone, can also cause VF. They, on occasion, cause a type of VT called *torsades des pointes* ("twirling around a point"). Several drugs used to treat ventricular arrhythmias such as sotalol, quinidine, procainamide, disopyramide, and lidocaine prolong the QT interval and aggravate or cause torsades, VT, and VF. Some drugs and other substances such as fluoxetine (Prozac), cimetidine (Tagamet), grapefruit and starfruit juice, and St. John's wort cause inhibition of a group of enzymes known as cytochrome P450 (CYP) that breaks down many drugs. This effect slows the breakdown of several drugs so that overdosing with these drugs can occur. When other drugs such as clarithromycin (Biaxin) and haloperidol (Haldol) are taken with the drugs and substances mentioned earlier, a prolonged QT interval can occur. This effect may be potentially dangerous as the person is placed at risk for ventricular arrhythmias.

People who use cocaine, amphetamines, methamphetamines, propofol, ket-amine, and other such drugs may die from VF as a result of the toxic effects on the heart. Often these drugs are taken together in combination and it is difficult to identify the specific drug that is the culprit. Some of these drugs cause both coronary artery spasm and direct damage to the heart muscle, making the heart especially susceptible to VF.

It is possible that Michael Jackson, River Phoenix, John Belushi, Jim Mor-rison, and Jimi Hendrix died from the cardiorespiratory effects of drug overdose. The exact cause of death is often not clear, though there was evidence of drug administration or usage in each case. Cardiopulmonary arrest is often caused by a combination of respiratory arrest, cardiac arrest, and aspiration of stomach con-tents into the trachea and lungs causing choking. It is likely that the arrhythmia causing death is VF, though definitive documentation is absent.

Dietary Causes

In the 1970s, very low calorie diets (VLCD) made from liquid protein consist-ing of hydrolyzed collagen and gelatin obtained from the bones and hooves of cows and horses were introduced. In the late 1970s, there was a spate of deaths caused by VLCD that resulted from heart muscle damage. Many of these deaths were due to VF associated with a long QT interval. The people who died were young, often in their twenties or thirties, and had lost about 35 percent of their body weight. These diets obtained from bovine and equine sources were deficient in micronutrients and amino acids, such as methionine, lysine, and tryptophan, which are necessary for the cellular integrity of heart muscle. These diets were banned by the Food and Drug Administration after dozens of deaths occurred in the 1970s and 1980s as a result of their use.

In 1988, when Oprah Winfrey declared on her television show that she had lost 67 pounds on a very low calorie diet, there was resurgence in the use of VLCD diets. All VLCDs promise weight loss, but at a cost as there are significant reductions in the intake of essential nutrients, which can lead to cardiac damage. Modifications of the original VLCD with added micronu-trients and essential amino acids are in wide use today. These newer VLCD must conform to the National Heart, Lung and Blood Institute guidelines that state that if they contain less than 800 kilocalories per day, they must also contain 70 to 100 grams of protein per day. This amount of protein is as-sumed to be protective of heart muscle damage. The European guidelines are very similar, though in the European Union countries (except France) VLCD products can be purchased over the counter with much less supervision than in the United States. To avoid cardiac death, such diets must be used under strict medical supervision, and regular EKGs must be done to monitor for QT-interval prolongation.

Some young women with anorexia nervosa are also at risk for cardiac death as they become deficient in these same amino acids. People going on extremely low-calorie diets should therefore check with their doctors because of the risk of sudden death.

Hypothermia

Extreme hypothermia can cause a variety of problems and the heart may go into VF during rewarming. Such cold hearts may be resistant to defibrillation. Special treatment protocols exist for rewarming for the treatment of people who fall into icy water, or are inadvertently exposed to extreme cold (e.g., when mountain climbing or when trapped in cars during the winter) to avoid cardiac arrest. Rewarming must be done very carefully according to protocol to avoid causing VF.

Trauma to the Chest

Traumatic blows to the chest may also trigger VF, as described earlier. This condition is seen usually in children as the chest cage is thin and trauma can directly affect the heart if the child is exposed to chest trauma. When a child falls from a tree or is hit on the chest by a baseball, tragically, death can occur if the strike occurs during the vulnerable period of the heart. A chest guard is recommended for protection during baseball games and some contact sports.

Electrocution

Household electric current can cause death from VF. In the Americas except Argentina the household standard is 120 volts and 50 or 60 hertz, while in Europe, much of Africa, and much of the rest of Asia, it is 220–240 volts and 50 hertz. Both systems can cause VF when a short pulse is delivered to the body and the jolt traverses the vulnerable period of the EKG.

Electricity is used for electroshock therapy (ECT) in psychiatrically depressed patients. This treatment is always done under anesthesia and with EKG monitoring and a cardiologist in attendance (specifically for high-risk cardiac patients). In some patients VF does occur and therefore a crash cart with a defibrillator and oxygen should always be on standby.

In cases of deliberately induced human death, drugs or electricity are used to terminate life. This happens when people commit suicide, in assisted suicide, and during judicial executions. Judicial execution is accomplished by using a lethal drug injection protocol. A combination of three drugs is given as a lethal injection: a barbiturate, a muscle paralyzing agent, and potassium. The barbiturate (sodium thiopental) causes loss of consciousness in less than a minute and depresses respiration when injected intravenously or intramuscularly. Pancuronium bromide (Pavulon) causes muscle paralysis and slows down breathing. A high dose of intravenous potassium chloride causes cardiac slowing and asystole, stopping the heart completely and causing death in a few minutes.

When electricity is used in the electric chair for judicial execution, a high voltage AC shock is administered via electrodes placed on a person strapped down in a chair. The Nebraska electrocution protocol of 2007 calls for the 20-second-long application of 2,450 volts of electricity. The shock may be repeated if the person does not die. The cause of death is complex and often not due to VF, but rather from paralysis of respiration and asphyxiation. There is extensive damage to internal organs from electrical trauma. In some cases, the person may actually catch fire and suffer extensive thermal skin burns.

Asystole

Cardiac arrest due to the heart stopping suddenly with absolutely no electrical activity is relatively unusual as a natural cause of human death. This condition, called *asystole*, is seen when there is total failure of the conduction system to generate any electrical activity. Asystole results from aging of the conduction system or from the effects of certain medications. As a person ages, the conduction system of the heart slows down and impulses from the atria are blocked from entering the ventricles. In other cases, the sinoatrial (SA) node stops firing, but the heart does not stop completely. This is because pacemakers situated lower in the heart (e.g., in the atrioventricular [AV] node or the ventricles) take over heart rhythm, but at a slower rate than normal. The heart stops completely if these lower pacemakers do not take over, and the only treatment that is effective is cardiac pacing.

Asystole can also be caused by massive pulmonary embolism when a very large clot travels to the main pulmonary artery trunk and blocks it almost completely. Not much blood can be pumped through such a large clot into the lung circulation, so that oxygenation is not possible. The heart then stops completely from lack of oxygenation. It is unlikely such a patient will survive unless the clot is surgically evacuated or treated with heparin and a thrombolytic agent to break up the clot. If such interventions are done rapidly, the patient may survive, but a large pulmonary embolism results in a high mortality rate.

The heart can become so heavily damaged during a myocardial infarction that it pumps very weakly. This leads to a condition called *electromechanical dissociation* (EMD) or *pulseless electrical activity* (PEA). In this situation, the electrical activity results in no mechanical contraction and blood is therefore not pumped out of the heart. This condition is very serious and most patients do not survive PEA. The heart eventually stops all electrical activity and comes to a halt in asystole.

DEFIBRILLATOR DEVICES

Though VF can abort spontaneously, especially in smaller animal hearts, it generally takes an electrical discharge to terminate this arrhythmia. Today, a variety of electrical devices that are collectively called *defibrillators* exist in different forms and they can effectively restore sinus rhythm. Though the different types of defibrillator in clinical use are basically similar, they are adapted for different clinical situations and designed to be used by different types of operators.

External Defibrillators

An external defibrillator is an electrical device that is capable of storing an electrical charge and discharging it through the chest wall or directly on the heart when needed. If successful, the shock restores the heart to a normal rhythm by terminating VF, and this process is called *defibrillation*. The basic electric circuit consists of a capacitor, an inductance coil, and a resistor. The defibrillator generates waveforms that are either a half-sinusoidal wave or a trapezoidal wave. In many devices, there is also a timing device incorporated in the circuit to allow a discharge that will synchronize with the R-wave of the EKG. This adaptation allows electricity to be used to revert arrhythmias other than VF (e.g., atrial fibrillation and atrial tachycardia). The process of reverting arrhythmias other than VF is called *cardioversion*.

The capacitor in an external defibrillator is charged from an AC wall socket or a self-contained battery, and the device typically charges up to 4,000 volts. The capacitor stores the energy until it is ready to be discharged. It takes about six seconds to charge to full capacity and a single DC pulse lasting approximately five milliseconds. The amount of the electrical discharge can be set as low as 10 joules and as high as 400 joules. A dial shows the amount of stored energy when the defibrillator is charged. The discharged energy is somewhat lower than the stored energy and indicators on the dial may also show the approximate energy that is delivered. Generally, a stored energy of 400 joules results in a discharged energy of 360 joules. The power control unit is connected to two chest electrodes or "paddles" by flexible cables.

The electrodes are covered with conductive paste and then placed on the chest in appropriate positions so that the discharge travels through the heart from the positive electrode to the negative electrode. Pre-gelled adhesive electrodes are also available for some types of defibrillators. The ideal positions for placement of the electrodes or paddles allows for the electrical discharge to envelope the heart. One electrode is generally placed at the right upper sternal border, and the second electrode is at the apex of the heart.

For VF, the maximum stored energy of 400 joules is usually used to defibrillate the heart. However, with highly trained operators, low-energy defibrillation using 100 joules is often done as this procedure reduces cardiac damage from electrical current. When the device is charged, pressing two switches simultaneously on the paddles triggers release of the electrical charge. During this time CPR should always be continued as it may take several minutes to get ready for defibrillation. Sometimes, even after discharge of the device, CPR has to be continued as the heart may not recover immediately and beat normally.

A defibrillator in a hospital setting is usually placed on a "crash cart" that is marked in red so that it is readily visible. Every intensive care unit, operating suite, emergency medicine department, and critical care area has at least one crash cart in place. The cart contains equipment for endotracheal intubation so that a doctor can insert a clear plastic tube into the throat using a laryngoscope. Various cardiac drugs, intravenous fluids, syringes, and needles for vein access are also stored in the cart. Most carts also have oxygen tanks and a breathing face mask for delivery of oxygen. The crash cart provides easy access to the defibrillator and vital accessory equipment needed for advanced CPR.

Automated External Defibrillators

Cardiac arrest occurs with no warning and, most often, in locations where there is no immediate medical help. Calling an ambulance, even in a large city in the United States, will take about 15–20 minutes at best before help arrives. To provide ready access to lifesaving technology, portable automatic defibrillators have been made available at public locations such as sports stadiums, airports, shopping centers, colleges, and large office buildings.

Automatic defibrillators are designed to be used by laypeople and require little training to be operated correctly. The automated external defibrillator (AED) units are based on computer-based algorithms and EKG technology designed to recognize patterns in order to analyze heart rhythms. Voice prompts advise the user whether a shock is required when VF or rapid ventricular tachycardia is recognized by the system. Functionally, AEDs are usually limited in their interventions to delivering high-energy shocks for VF and VT.

The automatic units take 10–20 seconds to analyze and diagnose the underlying rhythm. A trained professional can diagnose and treat the condition far more quickly with a manual unit, and if one is available, this device should be used rather than an AED. The longer time intervals for analysis, which require stopping chest compressions, have been shown in a number of studies to have a significant negative effect on treatment success. This effect led to the recent change in the American Heart Association defibrillation guidelines, calling for two minutes of CPR after each shock without waiting to analyze the cardiac rhythm, so as to provide circulation. Some organizations recommend that AEDs should not be used when manual defibrillators and trained operators are available.

Implantable Defibrillators

The defibrillator has been miniaturized to the size smaller than a cell phone, and is implanted in the front of the upper chest. Implantation of an ICD is done under local anesthesia. The device is connected to electrical cables (electrodes) threaded into the heart via a vein under the collarbone. Implantable defibrillators are discussed in full in Chapter 9.

Wearable External Defibrillators

In some patients who seem to meet the criteria for implantation of an ICD, it is not always clear whether they should have the procedure performed as it is unclear if permanent implantation will be of benefit. In some cases, the patient may simply refuse implantation of a device. When treating patients with severe muscle disease who are awaiting a transplant, there is a risk of sudden death. Some patients may have an infection that prevents immediate implantation of a device as the ICD may become infected as well. In these cases, a wearable external defibrillator may be of value. Wearable defibrillators are discussed in Chapter 9.

CARDIOPULMONARY RESUSCITATION (CPR)

The first section in this chapter focused on advances in cardiac revival from cardiac arrest. Much of the knowledge about how to do CPR evolved as a result of understanding how cardiac arrest actually happens and should be treated. This section focuses on CPR done mainly by bystanders and people who have been trained to give initial support at the beginning of a cardiac arrest. Such early treatment improves survival though overall survival rates following cardiac arrest are still very low.

Because more than 300,000 cardiac arrests occur annually in the United States in homes and in public places, such as shopping malls, stadiums, train stations, or airports, this is an important public health issue. As this problem is a widespread issue, everyone should be trained in the basics of CPR, as a relative or friend may collapse and die in a variety of private and public locations.

What Is CPR?

The term cardiopulmonary resuscitation (CPR) refers to the use of chest compressions and artificial ventilation by another human being to maintain blood flow and oxygenation during cardiac arrest. There are three basic levels of CPR:

A. Basic Life Support (BLS)
   Bystander CPR is delivered by laypersons who are trained in the basics of chest compression, airway maintenance, and ventilation support.
B. Advanced Life Support (ALS)
   This form of CPR is given by specially trained medical personnel who use defibrillators and medications.
C. Pediatric Advanced Life Support (PALS)
   For children, advanced life support has different guidelines from those for adults.

Details on CPR for laypeople can be found at this site of the American Heart Association: www.heart.org/cpr.

Since 92 percent of people with cardiac arrest die before reaching the hospital, it is important for bystanders to learn CPR as it can save lives. Though the rate of survival is dismally low at this time, rapid response times, innovations in treatment to protect the brain and new medications will hopefully increase survival rates in the future.

How Is CPR Done?

For a long time, CPR was taught with an acronymic "A–B–C" sequencing. This meant that the bystander did three things as follows:

A. *Airway check:* Make sure there is no obstruction in the throat. Open the mouth, pull the chin back, and allow the pharynx (throat) to open. This ensures that the larynx and upper trachea straighten out and connect with the upper throat with no kinking.

B. *Breathing:* Blow into the mouth rapidly and repeatedly to inflate the lungs. This delivers oxygen to people when they are not breathing on their own.

C. *Chest compression:* It is recommended that you check the neck (carotid) pulse right at the beginning, before the airway check, to see if there is a pulse. This establishes if the person is in fact in cardiac arrest before starting CPR. Once the airway check is done and assisted breathing is established, you start chest compressions.

Many people are afraid to put their mouths on a stranger's mouth and blow air directly into the lungs, for hygienic reasons. However, it has also been recently discovered that chest compression alone works well and gives satisfactory results. This variation of CPR known as "hands-only" or "compression-only" CPR (COCPR) consists solely of chest compressions and is effective in reviving a person.

The 2010 revisions to the American Heart Association CPR guidelines state that untrained bystanders should perform COCPR in place of standard CPR. The guidelines are summarized below:

A. The sequence of steps has changed from "A–B–C" (airway, breathing, chest compression) to "C–A–B" (chest compressions, airway, breathing). This applies only to adults and not to newborns.

B. The compression depth for adults should be at least two inches.

C. The compression rate should be at least 100 times a minute.

D. Defibrillation (if indicated) along with post-cardiac arrest care in a hospital facility.

It is more important to provide circulation with chest compressions rather that to provide immediate ventilation. This is because stopping compressions, even to give just two breaths, causes blood flow to stop. The cessation of blood flow leads to a quick decline in blood pressure despite the pressure built up during the previous set of compressions. Stopping compressions in order to provide ventilation is thus detrimental to the patient. However, straightening the neck to clear any obstruction should be done to prevent the tongue from falling back and causing the patient to choke.

CPR in the Community

Out-of-hospital cardiac arrests occurring in public areas are most likely to be associated with VF or rapid VT without a pulse. Such cases have better survival rates than arrests that occur at home. The reasoning is that CPR is often done by a group of bystanders and help often arrives more quickly to a public place. However, despite rapid response, application of advanced technology, and administration of cardiac drugs, survival rates are surprisingly low.

For out-of-hospital cardiac arrest the survival rate is less than 10 percent, and for in-hospital events, lower than 20 percent. Survival rates may be higher in men, but neurologic outcomes are better in younger people. Survival from cardiac arrest decreases by 10–15 percent for each minute of delay without CPR during cardiac arrest. This has led to the urgency of delivery of bystander CPR initiated within minutes of the onset of arrest to improve survival. Bystander CPR improves survival rates by two or threefold and also reduces neurological damage to the brain.

Indications for CPR

CPR should be performed immediately on any person who collapses, becomes unconscious, and is found to have no pulse. If there is no pulse, it means that the person may be experiencing cardiac arrest or may actually be dead. In other cases, the heart may not have stopped completely, but may be beating ineffectively and not pumping out blood. This situation occurs during VF, pulseless VT, or asystole. In some cases, there is no pulse though the EKG may actually show a normal rhythm. Such a condition, as already described above, is called *electromechanical dissociation* or *pulseless electrical activity* (PEA).

CPR should be started immediately if there is no pulse. Even in hospital, CPR is started (though an EKG machine may be available) before the rhythm is accurately identified. Electrical shock to defibrillate the heart should be applied as soon as possible if VT and VF occur. The more quickly the shock is applied, the greater the chance of terminating VF and subsequent full recovery. Additionally, CPR should be resumed immediately after a shock is administered and until a pulse is detected. Once the patient is stabilized with an airway and a normal rhythm established, he should be transported to an intensive care unit where further monitoring and treatment can be given.

Neurological Damage from Cardiac Arrest

The cells in the body most sensitive to lack of oxygen supply are brain cells. If the circulation stops for more than five to six minutes, irreversible cell death occurs. Thus, it is imperative that CPR be done as soon as cardiac arrest is detected. If defibrillation is done, chest compressions must be started again after the shock is administered, as normal circulation may take some time to be established even if the heart resumes beating normally. In other cases the first shock does not revert VF to a normal rhythm, so it is vital to continue CPR until a strong pulse can be detected.

Full recovery from cardiac arrest is possible if CPR and defibrillation are done rapidly. If CPR is prolonged, there is brain damage on recovery. Signs of brain damage include confusion, loss of memory, sleep disturbances, disorientation, loss of impulse control, inappropriate behavior, paranoia, and outbursts of rage, anger, and violence. Psychiatric counseling is necessary in such cases and medications may be needed to help the condition.

Besides rapid response in order to reestablish spontaneous circulation by advanced life support, whole body cooling has been tried to reduce the effects of brain damage. In patients who remain comatose after cardiac arrest due to brain damage, induced hypothermia may help recovery. Normal body temperature is 37 degrees Celsius or Centigrade (98.6 degrees Fahrenheit). Cooling the body with a special mattress with a cover delivering cool air, and with ice packs, reduces body temperature to 32–34 degrees Centigrade (90 to 93 degrees Fahrenheit). This process of cooling was found to reduce brain dysfunction and improve survival at six months. Both brain dysfunction and death rates were roughly 15–20 percent lower in patients who underwent body cooling. Infusions of crystalloid have also been used to cool core body temperature as it is more efficient, but this is still somewhat experimental. Further research in this area is required in order to improve survival from cardiac arrest.

Neurological complications occurring during cardiac arrest and following resuscitation are important because the amount of brain damage determines whether life support should be continued or terminated. Brain dysfunction is a key determinant in making end-of-life decisions.

Contraindications to CPR

Clinically, the only real contraindication to CPR is a written do-not-resuscitate (DNR) order by a doctor or an advanced directive document indicating a person's desire to not be resuscitated. Increasingly, people are aware they may develop brain damage during a prolonged resuscitation in the event of cardiac arrest. Some patients may simply feel that cardiac arrest is a quick and relatively painless way to end their lives as their time has come. If they have communicated their wishes to their loved ones, these wishes should be respected, even is there is no written documentation to support this position. If no DNR order is available, the doctor makes a decision during resuscitation based on the probability of recovery and may thus stop CPR. However, as far as possible, there should be full communication with relatives and loved ones to avoid anger and possible litigation. It is not a common occurrence, but some hospitals in the United States are allowing relatives and loved ones to be present during CPR so that they are not excluded and can witness the efforts made to revive the person.

A relative contraindication to performing CPR arises if it is judged that the delay in getting help has been so long that resuscitation would be medically futile because extensive brain damage has already occurred. If the patient has a severely disabling disease (e.g., terminal metastatic cancer), doing CPR is not going to change the prognosis. Such a decision may have been made beforehand or after the cardiac arrest has already occurred. This is a complicated medical decision that requires expert opinions and discussions with the family. Such a discussion avoids misunderstandings and second-guessing the medical decision-making process. Including the family is always a good idea as these situations are highly emotional and fraught with the danger of serious misunderstandings.

SUMMARY

Resuscitation from cardiac arrest is one of the great successes of modern scientific medicine. It is based on over 200 years of systematic observation, experimental research, and trial and error. Understanding how the heart works both as a mechanical and as an electrical organ was necessary before successful advanced CPR was discovered as a clinical treatment.

The development of the defibrillator has led to the revival of people who would otherwise be dead. For the first time in history, the dead can really be revived, and with both CPR and the availability of defibrillators in the community, chances of survival are improved.

12

Risk Factors for Coronary Heart Disease and Preventive Strategies

Case Study

James M., a 31-year-old pipe fitter who also played bass guitar in a rock band, had insulin-dependent diabetes since the age of 6. Due to failing kidney function as a result of diabetes, it was likely that he would develop renal failure, and eventually would need a kidney transplant. For this reason, he needed a pretransplant cardiac evaluation. Though he looked fit and healthy, he had high blood pressure and reduced pulses in his feet, suggesting poor circulation due to peripheral vascular disease. His vision was already failing from retinal hemorrhages due to diabetes.

Upon examination he looked pale and his pulse rate was 72 beats per minute, and his blood pressure was high at 160/100 millimeters of mercury (mmHg). His heart examination was normal and lungs were free of any fluid congestion. The remainder of his physical examination was normal.

The electrocardiogram (EKG) was also normal. His kidney function tests showed a high level of creatinine (3.5 milligrams per deciliter of blood [mg/dL] with the normal range being 0.5 to 1.2 mg/dL). The cholesterol blood test showed a high total cholesterol of 230 mg/dL, and a low-density lipoprotein (LDL) cholesterol of 160 mg/dL, which was also high. He was given a statin drug that lowered the LDL cholesterol to 90 mg/dL. He was treated for high blood pressure with medication, but a year later his kidneys failed due to diabetes and high blood pressure. As a result of increasingly poor vision and kidney failure, he had to quit working and give up his musical career.

James underwent kidney transplantation with an organ from a cadaver. The kidney functioned normally for the first several years and his blood pressure improved. Though he got married soon after I saw him, he and his wife separated two years after his transplant, and he lived alone in his own apartment.

Over the next five years, he developed anginal chest pains, difficulty in breathing, progressive peripheral arterial disease, and progressive eye damage due to diabetes. Eventually, he became legally blind. His diabetes was never really under control as he lived alone and did not eat regularly or follow a proper diabetic or low-fat and low-cholesterol diet. On occasion he would drink quite a bit, though he had cut back greatly on alcohol intake.

After he developed a severe episode of shortness of breath and angina, he underwent coronary angiography that showed three-vessel coronary artery disease. After heart surgery with three-vessel coronary bypass surgery, he made a good recovery. His angina was controlled and he seemed to improve. He then developed calf pain and a nonhealing foot ulcer due to peripheral vascular disease, eventually resulting in an amputation of the right leg below the knee. He was fitted with a prosthetic right leg, and he became largely wheelchair-bound.

After a cardiac arrest that occurred while visiting his mother, he was brought in unconscious to the emergency department and then admitted to the intensive care unit. After several days on a respirator, it did not seem he would recover. A computed tomography (CT) scan of the head showed an extensive stroke involving the left hemisphere of the brain. His transplanted kidney started to fail and dialysis was started. He did not breathe on his own, when he was taken off the respirator briefly to determine if he had spontaneous breathing. A repeat CT scan showed a larger area of infarction and an electroencephalogram suggested extensive brain damage.

At this point, we had a family conference to discuss his condition. It was decided jointly by the family and the medical staff that the respirator should be discontinued to allow him to die. The family gathered around with a priest in attendance, and after prayers and final Catholic rites, the respirator was turned off. He died a few minutes later. James was only 41 years old, but looked much older at the time of his death.

According to the World Health Organization, cardiovascular disease (CVD) causes 17.5 million deaths every year. CVD—heart disease and stroke—is responsible for half of all deaths in the United States and other developed countries. In rapidly industrializing countries, such as India, China, Brazil, Argentina, and Mexico, CVD is a major cause of death as well. Since these countries are shifting their economies from a predominantly agrarian base to industrial production, there are the accompanying stresses and strains of work, changes in dietary habits, exposure to atmospheric pollution, and alterations in social relations. These factors play a role in the increased rates of heart disease and stroke.

In the United States, more than 80 million Americans suffer from some form of CVD. Heart disease is the leading cause of death accounting for 29 percent of all deaths in 2007. Stroke, the third most frequent cause of death, accounted for 6.8 percent of all deaths in the same year. About 2,400 people die every day of CVD (heart attacks and strokes), accounting for half of all deaths in the United States. Cancer, the second largest killer, accounts for a little more than half as many deaths.

Coronary artery disease (CAD) is the most common cause of CVD, and it leads to about 1.2 million cases of myocardial infarction each year in the United States. According to the American Heart Association, over 7 million Americans have survived a myocardial infarction. About 25 percent of the people who suffer a heart attack (myocardial infarction and/or cardiac arrest) will die in an emergency department, or even before reaching the hospital. The economic burden of CVD to the United States is considerable and in 2010, CVD cost the nation $316 billion.

While the causes of heart disease are better understood and studied in more detail than with any other disease, our understanding of heart disease is still a work in progress. As with any disease, the main questions to be answered are twofold:

1. What are the causes of the condition?

and

2. What can be done to prevent the disease process?

Many theories have been proposed for the origin of CAD and several *risk factors* have been identified. Some alleged risk factors, such as the so-called *Type A Behavior* pattern, have been found to have only the most flimsy of connections to the onset of coronary atherosclerosis. In fact, in about half the cases, the actual underlying cause of coronary heart disease may not actually be found. In other words, not a single identifiable risk factor can be found in many cases, opening the possibility that there may yet be unidentified risk factors for CAD.

Furthermore, even when preventive measures are undertaken it does not necessarily mean that one will not eventually succumb to heart disease. The term *prevention* without further clarification is, therefore, a somewhat misleading term, if it is not properly qualified. What it simply means is that *preventive measures* act to delay the *early* or *premature onset* of heart disease. What prevention really means is the cardiac event is postponed to a later time in the person's life, and it does not mean that the person will *never* have a heart attack. Aging will eventually result in some degree of coronary artery disease, even if one has normal cholesterol levels, normal blood pressure, or a perfect genetic profile. There are, however, certain *risk factors* for early development of heart disease, and this chapter will describe them. Strategies for the prevention of the premature onset of heart disease will also be discussed.

CONCEPT OF RISK FACTORS FOR CORONARY HEART DISEASE

The Framingham Study

In the town of Framingham, Massachusetts, in 1948, a joint research project was started between the National Heart, Lung and Blood Institute and Boston University. Framingham, a town 21 miles west of Boston, was selected as a typical middle-class "Middletown USA" community to serve as a study population for heart disease. It was the hometown of Crispus Attucks, the first casualty who was shot dead by British Redcoats in the Boston Massacre of 1770. Though larger and wealthier today, Framingham remains a relatively small town with 67,000 people as of 2007. Though it is ethnically more diverse today, it still has a predominantly white population of 80 percent, with 10 percent Hispanics, and 5 percent each of African Americans and Asians.

The objective of the Framingham Heart Study (FHS) was to identify the factors that contribute to CVD by following its development over a long period of time in a large group of participants. Within the cohort were participants who had not yet developed clinical symptoms of CVD or already suffered a heart attack or stroke. Early preventive strategies have been devised based largely on the results of the FHS. Several other studies have since been conducted in Minnesota, Britain, Sweden, and other countries, to identify factors that increase the risk of coronary heart disease and myocardial infarction.

The FHS researchers initially recruited 5,209 men and women between the ages of 30 and 62. They conducted interviews on lifestyle, performed physical examinations, and drew blood for cholesterol and other tests. For over 60 years, since 1948, the study subjects continued to return to the study every two years for a repeat medical history, physical examination, and laboratory tests. A second group of 5,124 people was enrolled in 1971. This second group was the original participants' adult children and their spouses, and they underwent similar examinations.

In April 2002, a third generation was enrolled. These participants were the grandchildren of the original group. This three-generation study is unique because it will enable researchers to understand how CVD is inherited and how family constellations affect the development of the disease. The initial phase of this part of the study was completed in 2005. It is hoped that the historical aspects, physical findings, and blood tests gathered from the participants will help unravel the complex factors that produce CVD and get at root causes. The aim is to collect data that will help understand how to diagnose, treat, and prevent CVD.

As a result of theses studies, the concept of *risk factors for coronary artery disease* emerged. These factors can be categorized as *major* and *contributory risk factors*. There is good evidence that the major risk factors, such as age, genetic predisposition, high cholesterol, smoking, and high blood pressure, play a role in causing heart attacks, leading to an early death. Other biological and psychosocial factors play a contributing role. These factors include alcohol, high homocysteine levels, and psychosocial attributes such as employment status, marital status, bereavement, depression, education, church going, psychological stress, and so on. However, it is not always clear how these factors are associated with higher rates of myocardial infarction or sudden cardiac death, or why such factors do not seem to act as a risk factor equally in all people.

MAJOR RISK FACTORS FOR CORONARY HEART DISEASE

Major risk factors are those conditions that can be statistically shown to be strongly linked to the occurrence of coronary heart disease (CHD). Some of these risk factors can be modified, treated, or controlled, while others cannot be controlled. Risk factors can be additive in their effect. The more risk factors a person has, the greater the chance of developing coronary heart disease. For example, the coexistence of both diabetes and high blood pressure increases the risk of CHD more than if either factor alone were present. If high cholesterol is added to the list, the risk of developing a heart attack at an early age increases even more. Table 12.1 shows the major risk factors for CHD and whether they can be treated or controlled.

Among American adults, over a third, or 37 percent, have one or more risk factors for CVD. The frequency of distribution of risk factors in the United States population is shown in Table 12.2.

Age, Sex, and Heredity

Major risk factors that cannot be changed are age, gender, genetics, and a family history of heart disease. Over 80 percent of people who die of coronary heart disease are over 65 years of age. Though women have a greater heart attack risk after menopause, they are still at lower risk than men. It is likely that estrogen has protective effects against heart attacks in women, but women who have heart attacks are more likely to die than men.

Children of parents with heart disease are more likely to develop the condition themselves. African Americans have more severe high blood pressure problems

Table 12.1 Major risk factors for coronary heart disease

Major Risk Factors	Can Be Treated or Controlled
Age	No
Heredity/race	No
Male sex	No
High cholesterol	Yes
High blood pressure	Yes
Smoking	Yes
Diabetes	Yes
Inactivity and obesity	Yes

Table 12.2 Percentage of U.S. adults with risk factors in 2005/2006

Risk Factor	%
Inactivity	39.5
Obesity	33.9
High blood pressure	30.5
Cigarette smoking	20.8
High cholesterol	15.6
Diabetes	10.1

Source: Centers for Disease Control and Prevention, Atlanta, Georgia.

than Caucasians, and also have a greater risk for developing heart disease. Heart disease risk is also higher among Mexican Americans, Native Americans, and Native Hawaiians. This is partly due to higher rates of obesity and diabetes. East Asian-American women have the lowest risk for CHD, and the percentage of deaths in different populations in the United States is shown in Table 12.3. Since heredity and family history cannot be changed, it is all the more important that other risk factors be controlled or treated.

There are many genetic factors that play a primary role in inherited diseases, such as familial hypercholesterolemia and diabetes. It is believed that genetic factors interact with environmental factors. This interaction is complex and poorly understood in many cases. It is likely that major risk factors interact with contributory factors that may be environmentally influenced to produce premature onset of CVD.

In families with a high prevalence of heart disease, and early death, it is strongly recommended that children and young adults be screened for CVD. Such screening will include the risk factors enumerated below. This approach allows doctors to recommend preventive strategies such as dietary management, exercise programs, and appropriate medical treatments, if necessary.

In November 2011, the American Academy of Pediatrics issued guidelines for screening and treatment for children with high cholesterol. The guidelines for treatment have met with criticism, as they suggest early treatment for asymptomatic children. Since the long-term toxicity of statin drugs in children is not known, the safety of prescription in asymptomatic children with moderately high levels of cholesterol is an open question. However, if the child is obese, has hypertension, or a has strong family history of heart disease or hypercholesterolemia, he or she should be screened beginning at age 10 and treated under guidance from a pediatric specialist.

Table 12.3 Prevalence of death from CAD in various ethnic groups in the United States

Race of Ethnic Group	Percentage of Deaths
African Americans	25.8
American Indians or Alaska Natives	19.8
Asians or Pacific Islanders	24.6
Hispanics	22.7
Whites	27.5
All	27.2

Source: Centers for Disease Control and Prevention, Atlanta, Georgia.

Cholesterol Profile

Cholesterol is a waxy substance found in plants and animals. It is a type of fat and part of a complicated system of *lipids* found in blood and tissues. Cholesterol is essential for life as it is required for normal cell membrane integrity and func-tion and all cells, therefore, contain cholesterol in the cell walls.

In the liver, cholesterol is converted to bile that is then stored in the gallblad-der. Bile contains bile salts, which are necessary for the intestinal absorption of fat molecules as well as for the fat-soluble vitamins (A, D, E, and K). Cholesterol is also the precursor for the synthesis of Vitamin D, and it is the basis for the synthesis of steroid hormones, such as cortisol and aldosterone, synthesized by the adrenal glands. The sex hormones testosterone, estrogen, and progesterone are all synthe-sized from a cholesterol base. It is clear that cholesterol is a vital substance for life, but an excess creates problems of atherosclerosis in the cardiovascular system.

Lipids, or fats, are carried in the blood by proteins and the combination is called a lipoprotein. High levels of *blood lipids* lead to a condition called *hyperlip-idemia* that promotes atherosclerosis and leads to CVD. In 1985, Michael Brown and Joseph Goldstein, both at Southwestern Medical Center in Dallas, were awarded the Nobel Prize in Physiology or Medicine in 1985 for their work on the functions of the LDL cholesterol receptor and how the liver processes LDL cholesterol. It is the lack of LDL receptors on liver cells that is responsible for the genetically inherited familial hypercholesterolemia.

Types of Cholesterol

There are two main types of cholesterol: *low-density lipoprotein cholesterol* (LDL) and *high-density lipoprotein cholesterol* (HDL). High levels of LDL are toxic to the lining of blood vessels and cause plaque formation. Thus LDL is colloqui-ally known as *bad cholesterol*. On the other hand, HDL cholesterol is protective against atherosclerosis and is known as *good cholesterol*.

Lipids and cholesterol can originate in the diet (exogenous) or in the liver through synthesis (endogenous). Only about 25 percent of cholesterol comes from the foods we eat. The other 75 percent is made by the liver. All animal fats contain some cholesterol and the main dietary sources are butter, cheese, egg yolk, pork, beef, and shrimp. Factors such as age and genetics affect how much cholesterol the liver makes. High levels of LDL cholesterol in the blood can lead to plaque formation inside arteries, and this buildup leads to heart attacks and strokes, as described earlier.

Trans fats are a group of unsaturated fats that raise LDL cholesterol and lower HDL cholesterol. Adding hydrogen to vegetable oils by an industrial process called hydrogenation creates trans fats, and this is how margarine is produced. This process was introduced to solidify oils and slow spoiling. Trans fats have been shown to accelerate the development of CVD because they raise LDL cholesterol. Foods that contain a good deal of trans fats include french fries, doughnuts, shortening, cake mixes, pie crusts, pizza dough, ramen noodles, stick margarine, and most fast foods. The American Heart Association recommends no more than 1 percent of total calories be made up of trans fats. That is to say, in a 2,000 calorie diet, no more than 20 calories should come from trans fats.

Symptoms

By itself a high cholesterol level produces no symptoms. However, in some people, depositions of cholesterol can be seen on the skin as *xanthomas*. These depositions on the skin are usually around the eyes, and on tendons around the fingers, elbows, and knees. The presence of xanthomas on the skin alerts the physician to the possibility that a person may have hypercholesterolemia. Symptoms are caused by cholesterol and fat creating plaque that obstructs blood vessels, leading to angina, myocardial infarction, and stroke.

Diagnosis

The presence of elevated lipids in the blood is called *hyperlipidema*, and the diagnosis is made with a blood test that can help predict the risk for heart disease. The blood test shows the level of the different types of cholesterol and fats in the blood. Food intake boosts the level of cholesterol and triglycerides in the blood and this can make the results unreliable. Therefore, blood levels for a cholesterol profile are *always* drawn in the fasting state to establish a reliable baseline and for comparison before and after treatment with medications.

Blood tests are based on the amount of three types of lipids in the blood:

- Low-density lipoprotein (LDL), or "bad" cholesterol
- High-density lipoprotein (HDL), or "good" cholesterol
- Triglycerides

High levels of LDL in the blood clog arteries, and this increases the risk of heart attack and stroke. High triglyceride levels may also be harmful under certain circumstances. On the other hand, HDL cholesterol protects against heart disease. Tables 12.4, 12.5, and 12.6 show the levels of total cholesterol, LDL and HDL cholesterol, and the corresponding risk for CHD.

Table 12.4 shows the levels of total cholesterol that pose a risk for heart disease. Generally, *total cholesterol* alone is only a crude estimate of risk for CVD and is useful only for initial screening, and not used as the final target for the treatment of hyperlipidemia. The preferred target is LDL cholesterol, as this is the substance primarily responsible for atherosclerosis.

Table 12.5 shows the levels of LDL cholesterol that are normal and abnormal. These blood levels are the ones that are used clinically to guide medical treatment in most cases of hypercholesterolemia.

Table 12.6 below shows the risk of heart disease associated with HDL or "good" cholesterol. Higher HDL levels are desirable, as low levels generally indicate increased risk for CVD. It is thought that HDL cholesterol attenuates the toxic effects of LDL cholesterol. However, it has not been shown that artificially increasing levels of HDL cholesterol with medications will protect against heart disease.

Treatment for High Cholesterol Levels

Cholesterol levels should be tested in the blood of young adults for general screening, and in childhood when there is a family history of familial hypercholesterolemia. Drug treatment should be started in adults if the levels are out

Table 12.4 Cholesterol levels and risk for heart disease

Total Cholesterol Levels	What It Means
Less than 200 mg/dL	Desirable
200–239 mg/dL	Borderline high risk for heart disease
240 mg/dL and above	High risk for heart disease

Table 12.5 LDL cholesterol levels and what it means

LDL Cholesterol Levels	What It Means
Less than 100 mg/dL	Optimal
100–129 mg/dL	Near optimal
130–159 mg/dL	Borderline high
160–189 mg/dL	High risk for heart disease
190 mg/dL and above	Very high risk for heart disease

Table 12.6 HDL cholesterol levels and what it means

HDL Cholesterol Levels	What It Means
Less than 40 mg/dL	High risk for heart disease
40–59 mg/dL	Less risk for heart disease
60 mg/dL and above	Desirable

of line with the guidelines recommended by the National Cholesterol Education Program (NCEP) of the National Heart, Lung, and Blood Institute (NHLBI). The treatment of asymptomatic children with isolated elevated cholesterol will be discussed later and is presently controversial and unsettled.

Statins

Treatment of high cholesterol is important when the levels are very high, when other risk factors are present, or when heart disease is already established. The medication of choice today is a *statin*, the first line drug for treating this condition. A statin is a powerful drug that works on the liver to prevent production of cholesterol by blocking an enzyme called *HMG-CoA reductase*. Statins were discovered in 1976 by a Japanese scientist, Akira Endo, who isolated lovastatin (marketed later as Mevacor) from the fungus *Aspergillus terre*. Several statins have since been discovered or synthesized, such as atorvastatin (Lipitor), simvastatin (Zocor), pravastatin (Pravachol), and fluvastatin (Lescol).

The NCEP has provided guidance for the treatment of people with and without heart disease. The normal upper limit of LDL cholesterol is 130 mg/dL. However, for people who have no known CVD and no risk factors, or just one risk factor, treatment with drugs should be started only if the LDL cholesterol is over 160 mg/dL. If there are two or more risk factors, treatment is started if the LDL cholesterol level is more than 130 mg/dL.

Early treatment is imperative in people with angina, diabetes, and those who have suffered a previous heart attack. This group of people should be treated with a statin medication when their LDL cholesterol is greater than 100 mg/dL with the goal to bring the level to below 100 mg/dL. Multiple studies have shown such treatments reduce the death rate from heart attack and ultimately prolong life. When these patients are treated with statins, there is a reduction in coronary events, revascularization procedures (bypass surgery or angioplasty), cardiac mortality, and total mortality. Such reduction ranges from 24 to 42 percent depending on the clinical trial and the particular endpoint that was measured. Similarly, strokes are reduced by 19–27 percent in patients who are treated with statin drugs. There is also some evidence that the size of atherosclerotic plaque inside arteries may decrease with statin treatment and thus reduce obstruction to blood flow.

It should be emphasized that dietary discretion, weight reduction, and a regular exercise program are as important as treatment with statins. It also does not mean that by taking a statin, one can indulge freely in consuming fatty and unhealthy foods, though many people "cheat" on their diets believing they are protected by their statin medication.

At the present time, there is little or no evidence that healthy people will reduce their risk for coronary disease by taking statins. There is a greater probability of side effects from the drugs as statins do have serious toxicity such as liver damage and muscle damage.

Niacin

An alternate drug for treating high cholesterol is *niacin*. Niacin is also known as vitamin B3 or nicotinic acid. It can be found in chicken, beef, liver, tuna, fish, leafy vegetables, avocados, broccoli, fruits and nuts, dates, whole grains, and legumes. Niacin lowers LDL cholesterol and triglycerides and increases HDL cholesterol. It is available as an over-the-counter drug under the brand names *Niaspan* and *Niacor*. However, it should be used under medical supervision and with close monitoring of cholesterol levels as the doses used for cholesterol control are very large and this can cause side effects. Niacin can also be used in conjunction with a statin to enhance its effects. Niacin causes flushing, palpitations, and rash in some people, and aspirin can be used to reduce these side effects. Because large doses of niacin may cause liver damage, liver enzymes need to be monitored on a regular basis as with statins.

Cholestyramine

This drug is another agent commonly used to treat high cholesterol levels. Cholestyramine is a resin that is not absorbed, and works by binding bile salts in the gut. Bile is manufactured in the liver from cholesterol and discharged from the gallbladder so that it can help with the digestion and absorption of fats. Much of the bile is reabsorbed by the gut into the blood and reused. However, when cholestyramine binds with it, bile is not absorbed, and as it is excreted in the stool. This process is called sequestration. Since bile is essentially prevented from reentering the circulation, the body has to use up blood cholesterol to manufacture more bile. This process leads to lower levels of circulating blood cholesterol.

The side effects for cholestyramine are not pleasant, and it can cause rather severe constipation. It also binds drugs such as tetracycline, penicillin, barbiturates, digoxin, estrogen, progestin, diabetes medication, warfarin, thyroid medication, thiazides, and so forth. Thus, such drugs lose their efficacy if cholestyramine is added to the mix of medications and dose adjustments may be necessary.

Cholesevelam

Like cholestyramine, this agent is also a second-line drug that is a bile acid sequestrant. Cholesevelam (WelChol, Cholestagel) is a polymer that binds bile acids and lowers cholesterol in the manner described above. This drug is used as an adjuvant to statins rather than as a primary drug to lower cholesterol, unless a patient cannot tolerate the latter.

Fibrates

These agents are fibric acid derivatives, consisting of gemfibrozil (Lopid), clofibrate (Atromid-S), and fenofibrate (TriCor). Such drugs activate an enzyme called lipoprotein lipase that eventually promotes a reduction in cholesterol level. They are second-line drugs that enhance the action of statins or are used when a patient cannot take a statin due to side effects. Clofibrate has been associated with increased gallstone formation and is seldom used now. The other two drugs are used more frequently in order to enhance the effects of statins if needed.

Ezetimibe

Ezetimibe (Zetia, Ezetrol) inhibits absorption of fat from the intestines, but it is not used for primary treatment for hypercholesterolemia. Ezetimibe is only rarely used by itself, but rather often compounded with simvastatin and marketed under the brand name Vytorin. In drug trials, this drug used alone reduces LDL cholesterol, but does not reduce cardiovascular events. It is, therefore, not a first-line drug to be used alone, but rather a supplemental therapy, or an alternative in cases where statins cannot be tolerated.

Liver Transplantation

In some cases of familial hypercholesterolemia liver cells cannot bind LDL cholesterol and properly metabolize it. Such patients have a genetic defect and have extraordinarily high levels of LDL cholesterol. In one remarkable case, a little girl, Stormie Jones, inherited two separate defective genes from her father and mother resulting in LDL levels of over 800 mg/dL.

Single gene inheritance for familial hypercholesterolemia occurs about 1 in 500 times. In this situation, patients develop premature heart disease in the fourth and fifth decades of life and they die relatively young. Double gene inheritance for familial hypercholesterolemia occurs more rarely, about 1 in 250,000 times, as in the case of Stormie Jones. Medications do not work in these cases, and myocardial infarction and death occur before the age of 20.

Stormie Jones developed CVD in childhood and had two coronary bypass operations as well as a mitral valve replacement by the age of six. The risk of dying before the age of 10 in such a case is very high. It was therefore decided by her cardiologists that her only real chance of survival was to have combined liver and heart transplants. She certainly needed a normal liver that could process and metabolize the LDL cholesterol. Stormie had the first combined heart-liver operation done in 1984 by Thomas Starzl (b. 1926), a pioneering transplant surgeon in Pittsburgh.

After transplantation, LDL cholesterol level declined a remarkable 81 percent from 988 to 184 mg/dL. A second liver transplant was done in 1990 due to hepatitis of the first liver transplant, but sadly she died later that year at the age of 13. This is a particularly dramatic treatment for a very serious problem that occurs rarely. The operation, incidentally, had to be approved by the Human Rights Committee of the Institutional Review Board at the University of Pittsburgh, where this daring and radical operation was performed. Due to the shortage of livers available for transplantation, and the cost of transplantation, it is likely that genetic manipulation would be a more realistic way of treating this condition in the future.

Smoking

Practically everyone knows that smoking tobacco increases the risk of lung cancer. However, many people do not realize that smoking also greatly increases the risk of CVD and peripheral vascular disease (PVD). When other risk factors (e.g., high blood pressure, a high cholesterol, or diabetes) are present, the risk for CVD in smokers increases even more dramatically.

More than 400,000 Americans and many millions more around the world die each year of smoking-related illnesses. Cigarette smoking causes about one in every five deaths from all causes in the United States each year. Here is the scope of all-cause mortality caused by smoking:

- 444,000 deaths annually
- 50,000 deaths per year from secondhand smoke exposure
- 270,000 deaths annually among men
- 174,000 deaths annually among women

Smokers' risk of developing CVD is up to four times that of nonsmokers, and the risk for sudden death is increased twofold. People who smoke cigars and pipes or chew tobacco also have a higher risk of death from coronary heart disease, but their risk is lower than that for cigarette smokers. Exposure to other people's smoke—secondhand smoke—also increases the risk of heart disease. Cigarette smoking also acts in concert with other risk factors (e.g., genetic) to greatly increase the risk for CVD.

Smoking increases heart rate and blood pressure because of the stimulants contained in tobacco. Nicotine is the main ingredient in cigarette smoke, but other chemicals such as tar and carbon monoxide are also extremely toxic to blood vessels. These chemicals constrict blood vessels, lead to injury of the smooth lining of these vessels (the *intima*), and accelerate atherosclerosis. The chemicals in tobacco smoke also affect levels of fibrinogen (a blood-clotting component) in the blood; this change increases the risk of blood clots and, in turn, leads to a heart attack.

Nicotine is about the most toxic legally available substance that can damage the heart and blood vessels. This substance is so toxic that stopping it will extend life by about six years on average. If there is one risk factor that can dramatically reduce the incidence of CVD, it is smoking. Stopping tobacco is the single most important factor that can be modified to significantly lower the risk for heart disease and stroke.

Smoking cessation can be achieved by entering a rigorous program to quit smoking, by hypnosis, or by taking medication prescribed by a physician. Bupropion (Welbutrin, Zyban, Voxra) is an antidepressant that is often prescribed and should be used under medical guidance.

High Blood Pressure

High blood pressure, or hypertension, is defined as a systolic pressure higher than 140 mmHg and a diastolic pressure above 90 mmHg. Hypertension increases the heart's workload by making it pump harder. This causes the ventricular muscle to thicken, enlarge, and become stiff. It also increases the risk of stroke, heart attack, kidney failure, and congestive heart failure.

Hypertension is a major health problem, especially because it has no symptoms and most people who have hypertension are unaware of their condition. In the United States, about 50 million people, or 25 percent of the total population, have high blood pressure. More than half of all Americans over the age of 65 have hypertension. Hypertension is more common in men than women, is present more often in older people, and is more common in African Americans than in Caucasians. Besides being age-related and having a familial tendency, there are endocrine or hormonal disorders that can cause hypertension. The treatment in such cases, once discovered, is straightforward and removal of the offending cause is curative. In the majority of cases, there is no known cause and the condition is known as "essential hypertension."

When high blood pressure coexists with obesity, smoking, high blood cholesterol levels, or diabetes, the risk of heart attack or stroke increases several-fold. The combination of diabetes and high blood pressure is an especially toxic one because it leads to eye damage, blindness, heart disease, stroke, renal failure, and peripheral arterial disease. This combination was seen in James, our patient described in the case study at the beginning of the chapter. Reduction in blood pressure with medications will markedly lower the risk for both heart disease and stroke.

Diets high in salt can aggravate high blood pressure as salt tends to cause the body to retain water in order to keep body fluids at the correct osmotic concentration. Retention of water tends to increase the volume of blood and this puts additional strain on the heart. When congestive heart failure develops, it is common to restrict salt for this reason. It is, therefore, important to restrict salt in the diet in order to better control high blood pressure. Physical exercise also has a long-term effect of lowering blood pressure.

People over the age of 18 should have their blood pressure checked at least every two years. As they grow older, it should be checked once a year to make sure it is lower than 140/90 mmHg. The pressure should be taken again if it is high to recheck it, in case it was temporarily elevated due to stress, caffeine intake, or any other factors. If blood pressure remains elevated, appropriate medications should be started and a diet and exercise program followed.

Medications used to treat hypertension fall into several categories due to their mode of action. There is a systematic approach to treatment that is well documented by the NHLBI and referenced at the end of this chapter. These drugs include diuretics, alpha and beta-adrenergic blockers, calcium blocking agents, angiotensin-converting-enzyme (ACE) inhibitors, and angiotensin II receptor blockers (ARB).

Inactivity and Obesity

Though inactivity and obesity are separate risk factors, they will be dealt with as one as they tend to go together and it is helpful to consider a combined approach. An inactive lifestyle is a risk factor for coronary heart disease. Regular, moderate-to-vigorous physical activity helps prevent heart and blood vessel disease. Generally, vigorous physical activity confers greater benefits, to the body and to health, than lower levels of activity, but that does not mean that all people should engage in intense physical activity to prevent the early onset of heart disease. Moderate exercise helps to prevent onset of heart disease, if done regularly. Physical activity can help control blood cholesterol, diabetes, and obesity, and help lower blood pressure.

Inactive people are not always obese, but activity does help reduce body fat if a person is overweight as it is often difficult to lose weight with a diet alone.

Adding an exercise program to a dietary plan makes it easier to maintain weight loss. People who have excess body fat (especially around the waist) are more likely to develop heart disease and stroke, even if they have no other risk factors. Excess weight increases blood pressure and thus leads to increased work stress on the heart. It also raises cholesterol and triglyceride levels while lowering HDL ("good") cholesterol levels. Overweight people are also more likely to develop adult-onset diabetes. Losing weight, therefore, helps reduce the risk for both heart disease and diabetes.

Diabetes

Diabetes is caused by a lack of the amount of insulin needed to metabolize glucose for powering muscles and all living cells. Diabetes seriously increases the risk of developing CVD, kidney disease, and stroke. All of these conditions lead to premature death. Even when glucose (blood sugar) levels are under control, diabetes increases the risk of heart disease and stroke, but the risks are even greater if blood sugar is not well controlled. About three-quarters of people with diabetes die of some form of heart or vascular disease.

There are two types of diabetes: Type 1 and Type 2. In Type 1 diabetes, there is a lack of insulin production due to the destruction of the pancreas, and daily injections of insulin are necessary to correct this condition. Type 1 diabetes, also known as insulin-dependent diabetes mellitus (IDDM), usually has its onset in younger age groups. The metabolic derangements caused by diabetes are extremely complex and cause changes in nerves and blood vessels that become gradually damaged over many years.

Patients with IDDM have early onset heart disease due to accelerated atherosclerosis. They also develop peripheral vascular disease leading to lack of blood flow, usually to the legs. Nerve damage leads to a lack of sensation in the legs (neuropathy) making the person susceptible to injuries of which they are unaware. These changes lead to the development of foot ulcers due to lack of blood flow to heal injuries resulting from trauma. In some cases, arterial bypass surgery is necessary to improve blood flow. In severe cases, foot or leg amputation is necessary for severe pain and nonhealing ulcers. Another complication is impotence in males due to nerve damage and lack of blood flow to the pelvic organs.

Our patient above, James, had IDDM, hypertension, and a high cholesterol level. These three risk factors all worked in combination to lead to kidney failure and promoted early onset of coronary disease and peripheral vascular disease. The result of this combined process had a devastating effect on his body as a whole. Unfortunately, he developed all the complications associated with diabetes: coronary artery disease, peripheral vascular disease, kidney failure, and blood vessel damage in the eyes, leading to blindness. It is necessary, because of the risk of developing these complications, to make absolutely sure that blood sugar control is achieved with the correct doses of insulin and an appropriate diet.

In Type 2 diabetes, also known as adult-onset diabetes mellitus (AODM), there is insulin production but the person is resistant to insulin. Therefore, there is a "relative" deficiency of insulin and blood sugar levels are not well controlled. The main cause of AODM is being overweight. Some patients have insulin resistance, so that higher doses of insulin are needed, as well as medications that stimulate insulin production. As with IDDM, all of the complications described can occur, albeit at a later age and with a lesser degree of severity. Patients need to follow a regular diet, follow an exercise program, and have their blood A1C levels checked to avoid vascular and other complications regardless of whether they have Type 1 or Type 2 diabetes.

Contributory Risk Factors for Coronary Heart Disease

Besides major risk factors, there are contributory risk factors that seem to play a role in leading to coronary heart disease. These factors play a role in some people but not others, so it is extremely difficult to know how to measure and evaluate their effects on the body. Currently, we do not have tools precise enough to accurately measure the contributory factors that may play a role in causing heart attacks and premature death. This is particularly true of factors such as psychosocial factors and psychological stress. Table 12.7 below lists some contributory risk factors and indicates whether they can be modified.

Table 12.7 Contributory risk factors for coronary heart disease

Contributory Risk Factors	Can Be Treated or Controlled
Psychological stress	Yes
Anger	Yes
High body mass index	Yes
Physical inactivity	Yes
Alcohol	Yes
Homocysteinemia	Probably
C-reactive protein	Unclear

Alcohol

The effects of alcohol on the body and the role of alcohol in causing heart disease or protecting against it must take into account its effects on the body as a whole. The relationship of alcohol to the heart is a complex one and depends on the dose of alcohol consumed. It is likely that alcohol provides a modest protective effect in terms of CVD, but it can also cause other types of problems such as heart muscle disease and arrhythmias.

Moderate alcohol consumption protects against heart disease by raising HDL (good) cholesterol and reducing plaque formation. Alcohol also has a mild anticoagulant effect on blood platelets, preventing clumping and clot formation. The risk of heart disease in people who drink *moderate* amounts of alcohol (an average of about one drink for women or two drinks for men per day) is lower than in nondrinkers. One drink is defined as 1.5 fluid ounces (fl oz) of 80-proof spirits (such as bourbon, Scotch, vodka, gin, and so forth), 1 fl oz of 100-proof spirits, 4 fl oz of wine, or 12 fl oz of beer. The reduction is in *total mortality* (not cardiac mortality), and it occurs in those who drink 1–2 drinks a day. In teetotalers and in heavier drinkers, total mortality is increased. A large number of other diseases are also increased in heavier drinkers, These diseases include stroke, pancreatitis, cardiomyopathy, atrial fibrillation, hypertension, cirrhosis, several kinds of cancer, as well as accidents, homicide, and suicide.

It's not recommended that nondrinkers start using alcohol or that those who drink currently increase the amount they consume. Drinking more than three drinks a day has a direct toxic effect on the heart. Heavy drinking, particularly over time, may lead to high blood pressure and damaged heart muscle resulting in *alcoholic cardiomyopathy*. In alcoholic cardiomyopathy, the heart muscle is damaged so badly that it cannot pump properly, leading to enlargement and congestive heart failure. Heavy drinking also delivers more fat into the circulation by raising triglyceride levels. Thus, consuming alcohol is not the best way to reduce heart attack risk. It is far better and healthier to reduce risk of heart disease by eating right, getting regular exercise, and maintaining a healthy weight.

Alcohol, incidentally, can also cause irregular heartbeats and is a frequent cause of *atrial fibrillation*. Binge drinking in college may lead to a frightening episode of fibrillation after an evening of partying (*holiday heart*). Older patients already have a higher incidence of AF due to aging of the heart. In susceptible patients, that nightly shot of whisky, brandy, or a cocktail may contribute to the development of atrial fibrillation. In atrial fibrillation, before embarking on drug treatment or invasive procedures such as electrical ablation of pathways in the heart, abstinence from alcohol should be attempted. Thus, despite alleged benefits of alcohol in protecting against coronary heart disease, the downside effects of alcohol, such as muscle damage and atrial arrhythmia, should also be considered.

Homocysteinemia

An amino acid called homocysteine can, in high levels, damage the inside lining of blood vessels. Though this is generally considered a risk factor for the development of CVD, lowering levels of homocysteine with folic acid, Vitamin B6, and Vitamin B12 does not reduce the risk of heart attacks. However, there is a 25 percent reduction in strokes with no reduction in mortality.

Homocysteine levels are generally not routinely monitored with a blood test for screening purposes by most cardiologists because the role of this chemical in atherosclerosis is not clear. An elevated homocysteine level occurring in the absence of CVD is not currently an indication for treatment. However, despite this uncertainly, many physicians have been prescribing folic acid for this condition anyway. In patients with CVD, currently, treatment with folic acid, Vitamin B6, and Vitamin B12 is recommended to lower homocysteine levels.

C-Reactive Protein

Another substance that is associated with a higher putative risk for CVD is C-reactive protein (CRP). High levels of CRP allegedly double the future risk for developing heart disease. It is not clear why inflammation results in high levels of CRP, but since it is part of the immune system, an increase during any illness may be part of a generalized reaction. The test has been popularized by Paul Ridker from the Brigham and Women's Hospital in Boston. Ridker and his collaborators conducted the multicenter JUPITER trial on 17,802 apparently normal people with normal cholesterol levels in the United States, South America, and Europe and published their results in 2008. Treatment with the statin drug rosuvastatin significantly reduced the incidence of CVD endpoints such as nonfatal myocardial infarction, stroke, and death.

The problem is that CRP is associated with many kinds of inflammation, such as rheumatoid arthritis, lupus, cancer, trauma, burns, and postsurgery. In 2009, Paul Elliott and his colleagues did a genetic association and replication study using Mendelian randomization on 31,582 people seeking a correlation between CRP and coronary heart disease. Their findings argue against a correlation of CRP with heart disease.

The main problem with the tests for both homocysteine and C-reactive protein is that an association between high levels of these chemicals and CVD is not proof of causality. More research is needed before definitive advice can be given to patients who have elevated blood levels with these substances present. The best that can be said is that if CRP is normal, the risk of a heart attack is low and that if CRP is high, one should treat the standard risk factors. There is no specific treatment for a high CRP.

Psychological Factors and Stress

The association between psychological factors, heart disease, and sudden cardiac death is part of the public imagination. Over the years many psychological factors have been suggested as risk factors for CHD and sudden cardiac death. Among these are the so-called Type A personality, anger, hostility, depression, bereavement, sleep deprivation, and lack of social networks. Despite the extensive amount of literature on this topic, risk factors such as Type A personality are too imprecise or inaccurate to be credible as definite risk factors for CAD. There seems, however, good evidence that factors such as depression significantly increase the risk for death, especially after a myocardial infarction. For example, in 1969 Colin M. Parkes in Great Britain showed that mortality for CHD was significantly increased in the first six months after the loss of a spouse. This effect is probably due to depression and loss of social support. While this effect was seen in both men and women, death rates were much higher in men than in women following conjugal bereavement. Anger and hostility have also been associated with a higher prevalence of angiographic evidence for CAD.

Life change events such as job loss, marital separation, divorce, imprisonment, retirement, and a total of 43 major social realignments measured by the Holmes-Rahe scale have been associated with various illnesses, including heart disease and sudden death. Whether factors such as depression, anger, loss of a job, or other significant life events actually accelerate the early development of CHD or precipitate a myocardial infarction and sudden death is not definitively known. Well-conducted studies show that the lack of social networks and the stress of conjugal bereavement are associated with increased incidence of coronary heart disease and cardiac death. However, a few studies have actually found no definite correlation between psychological factors and coronary heart disease.

The difficulty in studying psychological stress is that it is subjective and cannot be properly measured. Research consists of interviewing subjects and recording their subjective assessment of their feelings. The measurement tools are not precise enough to accurately quantify the extent of stress a person experiences and biochemical correlates are too variable even in the same subject for definitive conclusions to be drawn. However, it is known that both prolonged and episodic intense psychological stress can result in hypertension, metabolic derangements, and cause increases in adrenaline. There are also physical changes in cardiac contractile function and electrical alterations in the heart with provocation of arrhythmias.

The clinical question, however, is how patients with heart disease undergoing psychological stress should be treated. Some studies have shown that treatment of psychological distress and depression with psychological support, counseling, and home visits significantly reduces the likelihood of premature death after a heart attack. Even if the links between CHD, sudden death, and psychological stress are not precise, it is appropriate for medical caregivers to offer support, counseling, and treatment to improve the general health of the patient. One finite gain of attention to psychological needs is that there is an overall health benefit to a patient already suffering from a serious illness. It is likely that alleviation of psychological stress will have a salutary effect on outcomes.

Body Mass Index

Body mass index (BMI) is a formula to assess body weight in relation to height. This formula gives a measure of body composition and has been shown to be an effective predictor of the amount of body fat. BMI is used as a measure of obesity and in the metric system, is calculated using the formula shown in Table 12.8.

Table 12.8 Body Mass Index (BMI) formula

$$\text{BMI (kg/m}^2) = \frac{\text{weight in kilograms}}{\text{height in meters}^2}$$

Table 12.9 shows the range for underweight, normal, overweight, and obese individuals. However, it should be recognized that there is some debate whether this measure is a reliable index to accurately indicate the health status of an individual.

Table 12.9 Ranges for BMI for adults

Body Composition	Body Mass Index (BMI)
Underweight	Less than 18.5
Normal	18.5–24.9
Overweight	25.0–29.9
Obese	Greater than 30.0

Despite debates over the validity of BMI, it is recognized that lowering of body weight in overweight people lowers blood pressure in hypertension, lowers LDL cholesterol and triglycerides, and lowers blood glucose in diabetes.

Medications and Drugs

Certain medications and drugs can cause myocardial infarction. The long-term use of oral contraceptives can accelerate atherosclerosis, coronary artery disease, and stroke. These agents can also cause hypertension, and side effects are aggravated if the patient is a smoker. Use of contraceptive medication continuously for more than six years, especially if combined with smoking, is a very serious risk factor for premature onset of CVD. Myocardial infarction and stroke may occur in such women in their 20s and 30s, and smoking in women taking contraceptive medication should be strongly discouraged as it further increases the risk. The effect on blood lipids and blood sugar depends on the amounts of estrogen and progestin present in the contraceptive. In general, those medications containing only progestin have the least adverse effects on lipids and blood glucose levels. Effects on HDL and LDL cholesterol levels depend on the relative amount of estrogen that is present in the formulation of the contraceptive.

Ephedra (*ma huang*) is a Chinese herbal medicine that contains ephedrine and was banned in 2003 by the FDA. This action was taken because myocardial infarction due to ephedra was reported in several cases. It is also likely that the substance causes strokes. This observation underscores the fact that herbal medicine and "naturally occurring" medications are not all equally safe.

Another agent associated with myocardial infarction and sudden death is cocaine. Repeated use of this illegal drug causes intense coronary spasm, myocardial damage, and cardiac arrest. Unlike the long-term effects of tobacco and high cholesterol, which cause coronary artery disease over years, the onset of a heart attack and death is very rapid, and can occur within an hour or less of taking cocaine. The risk of a heart attack increases by over 24 times in people who take cocaine. The average age of the victim is also 17 years younger than the typical heart attack patient, so most victims are in their 20s and 30s. Most of the patients have no prior history of heart disease. Obviously, there is little to recommend the use of cocaine as a recreational drug, though many people still view it as such.

PREVENTION OF CVD

As mentioned at the beginning of this chapter, strategies for the *prevention* of CVD will not result in the total disappearance of CVD and its consequences, but rather progression of coronary artery disease is slowed and delayed. People are often astonished when they experience a heart attack with no prior known risk factors. We need to remember that heart and blood vessels will still age, even with normal cholesterol, lean body weight, normal blood pressure, and absolutely no risk factors. Besides aging, there may be yet unidentified risk factors that promote the development of CVD.

What is known is that 25 percent of people in the United States over 50 have at least two major risk factors for heart disease, with 80 percent of women aged 40–60 who have one or more risk factors for heart disease. Only 10 percent of the population has every risk factor under good control. Having just one risk factor doubles the chance of developing heart disease. What is not yet understood is what other unknown risk factors exist in those who appear to have none of the identified risk factors.

There is very good evidence that taking prudent steps can reduce the early onset of CVD and heart attacks. Large-scale studies that followed on the heels of the Framingham Study showed that interventions such as exercise, dietary management, and statin treatment reduce the incidence of myocardial infarction and death. Preventive guidelines have been generated by organizations such as the American Heart Association and the American College of Cardiology. These guidelines are classified as *primary prevention* and *secondary prevention*.

Primary Prevention of Heart Disease

Primary prevention consists of steps taken to reduce the impact of risk factors before there are signs and symptoms of CVD, and the disease becomes established. The aim of primary prevention also refers to the efforts to prevent the development of risk factors by a healthy lifestyle with the aim of delaying or preventing new-onset CVD.

Many of the primary prevention steps employed to prevent early onset of heart disease have already been discussed above. Basically, primary prevention refers to a healthy lifestyle consisting of dietary management, exercise, body weight maintenance, and avoidance of smoking or smoke-filled environments. Medication is part of primary prevention when there is hypertension, diabetes, and high cholesterol. In some older patients who are at high risk for CVD, aspirin can be considered part of primary prevention if it is administered.

Role of Exercise

Increased physical activity and aerobic exercise have long been shown to prevent coronary heart disease. Exercise has numerous beneficial effects. It strengthens the heart and improves physical endurance by increasing efficiency of oxygen use by muscles. Exercise increases energy level, lowers blood pressure, improves joint flexibility and balance, strengthens muscle and bone, and reduces body fat. Exercise also reduces stress, tension, and depression, and makes one feel more relaxed. In patients with heart disease, strengthening the contractile function of the heart helps alleviate symptoms such as shortness of breath. A full exercise program is available from the American Heart Association website.

Role of Antioxidant Vitamins

Oxidation is a chemical process that transfers electrons from a substance to an oxidizing agent. This process releases chemicals called *free radicals* that can damage cells. *Antioxidants* are agents that remove those free radicals, and reduce oxidative stresses that damage blood vessels and cause heart and vascular disease. It also seems that cancer is promoted by oxidative stress.

Allegedly, dietary supplements such as Vitamins A, C, and E and coenzyme Q10 act as antioxidants. These supplements are touted as reducing cancer and heart disease, but to date, there are no clinical or experimental data to support this case. In the case of coenzyme Q10, the National Institutes of Health has stated that it is "possibly effective" (though controversial) in helping manage congestive heart failure in combination with other drugs, but not by itself. There is weak evidence that coenzyme Q10 may reduce future recurrence of myocardial infarction if given early on during an myocardial infarction and that it reduces blood vessel damage during cardiac surgery. However, the evidence is not compelling enough to routinely treat such patients with this agent while they are hospitalized. There is no evidence that self-medication with coenzyme Q10 at home is helpful for any cardiac condition.

In fact, there is some suggestion that excessive use of antioxidants may cause harm. However, a diet rich in natural antioxidants, such as fruits, vegetables, whole grains, and nuts is a more sensible approach for reducing the risk of CVD. The American Heart Association does not recommend the addition of antioxidant supplements to prevent heart disease.

Role of Diet in Reversing Coronary Heart Disease

Dieting is something of a fashion industry. Every few years, both sensible diets and bogus diets with catchy names emerge and are heavily promoted on television. However, some reliable studies do suggest that once CAD is established, plaque can be reversed and blockages partially relieved by severe dietary restriction of fats and cholesterol. There are examples of brand-name diets such as the Pritikin and Ornish diets that sell packaged food to their clients. Though such diets probably do indeed reverse some degree of blockage and relieve symptoms of angina, the extreme restriction of fatty foods is difficult to maintain on a long-term basis.

Patients report improved well-being with severe restriction in animal fat and oils, but many patients ultimately relapse into past eating habits. Therefore, it would seem prudent to stick to a regular diet low in starches, fat, and cholesterol. This diet is the best option for long-term prevention of heart disease and for maintenance of a healthy lifestyle. A dietitian's guidance on a sensible and realistic diet is a far better option.

Role of Fish Oils

Unlike animal fats and trans fats, fish oils from fatty fish, like halibut, salmon, tilefish, swordfish, and tuna, seem to protect against heart disease. The main ingredient in fish oils is *omega-3* fatty acids. The fish do not actually make the omega-3 fats but accumulate them by eating algae or preying on other fish that have already accumulated such oils.

The beneficial effects are supposed to occur from reducing platelet stickiness, lowering triglycerides, and preventing ventricular arrhythmias responsible for sudden death. The current American Heart Association recommendation is to eat at least one gram of fish oil a day, or two servings of fish per week. Fish oil can also be consumed by taking fish oil capsules, which can be obtained without prescription from stores.

Secondary Prevention of Heart Disease

Secondary prevention refers to treatments to reduce the recurrence of CVD events and decrease coronary mortality in patients with established CVD. The presence of CVD is demonstrated by the occurrence of angina pectoris, myocardial infarction, history of coronary artery procedures (bypass graft or angioplasty), peripheral artery disease, and aortic aneurysm. Secondary prevention strategies are therefore aimed at both the control of risk factors, as well as direct therapeutic interventions that protect coronary arteries from plaque formation.

There is some overlap between actual treatment of CVD and secondary prevention, as the strategy and medications used are similar in both cases. So what is the difference between actual treatment for CVD and secondary prevention? The distinction is that after treatment of the acute event that brought the person to the doctor in the first place, a maintenance program is necessary to prevent progression of CVD, recurrence of myocardial infarction, and early death. The reason, simply, is that once someone has any of the cardiac or vascular events mentioned above, he or she is definitely at very high risk for developing another acute coronary event. Aggressive preventive measures are thus mandatory for prevention of a recurrent event. For purposes of secondary prevention, the American Heart Association has published recommendations for risk management in patients with established CVD. These guidelines are summarized at the end of this chapter.

The question may well be asked, does risk factor modification make a difference to health outcomes? The answer is a resounding "Yes!" There is plenty of evidence that suggests death rates from both coronary disease and CVD of all other types have been reduced by a better understanding, and therefore modifying behaviors. From 1979 to 2003, coronary heart disease decreased, from 333 to 177 out of 100,000 people, and other types of heart disease declined from 92 to 59 out of 100,000 people in the same period. Other types of CVD, such as peripheral vascular disease, stroke, and so forth, declined from 142 to 87 out of 100,000 people in that time frame.

The reason for the decline in all types of CVD is that there has been the development of better diagnostic methods, better drug treatment, safer and better surgical treatment, and increased risk factor modification. In fact, the most powerful of all interventions is risk factor modification and medical treatment with aspirin, beta-blockers, cholesterol-lowering drugs, regular exercise, and dietary modification, which have shown the most powerful effect on outcome after a myocardial infarction.

Cardiac rehabilitation following myocardial infarction and coronary bypass surgery is a structured approach to secondary prevention. Rehabilitation over a period of 12 weeks is done with exercise and dietary guidance to orient the patient to the process of recovery from the cardiac event. The effects of secondary prevention outweigh the effect of direct interventions on the heart such as angioplasty, stenting, and coronary bypass surgery. Though the latter interventions are more dramatic than secondary prevention, they are not as powerful as risk factor modification in reducing death from cardiovascular diseases.

Cardiovascular Disease in Women

Gender Differences

Much evidence suggests that there is a difference between men and women in cardiovascular responses to environmental and psychological stress. For example, women react to psychological stress with greater changes in heart rate and blood pressure. For many years, it was not recognized that men and women were not equally affected by CVD, nor was it apparent that symptoms and outcomes of CVD were dissimilar. In the past three decades, it has also become clear that women and men do not have the same clinical presentations, and that diagnosis may be delayed in women.

The net result is that over time the mortality rate for women has remained relatively flat compared to the rate for men, which declined steeply from 1979 to 1993. This trend is worse for African-American women than for Caucasian women, with deaths from CVD about 70 percent higher in that population. Trends seem to be similar for Hispanic women, though statistics are not as easily available. The higher death rates in African Americans and Hispanic women may be due to less fortunate economic circumstances, detection bias, lack of access to care, competing priorities, and errors in reporting.

In 2000, over 50 million American women were over the age of 50. Since incidence of CVD increases with age, CVD deaths for women are actually higher. The most common diagnosis for women upon discharge from a hospital is CVD (not breast cancer or any other disease associated with women). In fact, CVD is the cause of death in 45 percent of women, which is greater than all causes of cancer combined.

Perhaps one reason for this relative neglect until recently in reporting the risk of CVD in aging women is that the risk of dying from CVD is much higher in men than for women at the same age. On average, women tend to be 10 years older than men when experiencing their first heart attack. In other words, the risk of dying from CVD for a 40-year-old man is the same as a 50-year-old woman. It may also be that more attention has been paid by both the medical profession, and by women themselves, to breast cancer than to heart disease. This is true, despite the fact that less than 40,000 women died from breast cancer in 2010, while 316,000 women—almost eight times as many—died from CVD. The odds of dying from breast cancer are 1 in 35, while there is a 1 in 2 chance of dying from heart disease or stroke in women.

Risk factors for CVD in men and women are very similar. The main reason why women are protected for about 10 years longer than men may be that estrogen apparently protects women against CVD. After menopause, the protective effect of estrogen ceases and the risk for CVD increases.

CVD and Hormone Replacement Therapy

From the early 1940s, women going through menopause were treated with hormone replacement therapy (HRT) coupled with estrogens or estrogen replacement therapy (ERT) to overcome the side effects of menopause. It was believed that such therapy would reduce irregular menses, vaginal symptoms, flushing, palpitations, osteoporosis, dementia, and the effects of aging. To a great extent, this move was also driven by drug marketing efforts. The agents used singly or in various combinations were estrogens, progesterone, and progestins, sometimes with the addition of testosterone. Such replacement therapy was also recommended for women who had surgical menopause due to removal of the ovaries for disease conditions.

The agents were given orally, intravenously, or topically through application to the skin vaginally. The general idea was to simulate "normal" hormonal balance. It should be emphasized that such treatment was done in a most unscientific manner with no evidence whatsoever that the medications had any beneficial effect. The possible risks of such treatment were not known at the time, and such treatment would not be allowed today under current Food and Drug Administration rules.

Several long-term studies have since assessed the effects of such replacement therapy. The Women's Health Initiative (WHI) study was conducted by the National Institutes of Health to study the effects of Prempro, a combination of estrogen and progestin. The core part of the study showed that women taking the drug had a higher incidence of breast cancer, heart disease, and strokes. The WHI findings were confirmed in a larger national study done in the United Kingdom, known as the Million Women Study, that studied the effects of HRT. The study reported that women taking estrogen alone were not at risk for heart disease, but had a higher risk for endometrial cancer of the uterus and ovarian cancer.

As a result of these findings, the number of women taking hormone treatment has declined over time. The Women's Health Initiative recommended that women with normal menopause should take the lowest possible dose of HRT for the shortest possible time, when clinical indications suggest a need for treatment. To summarize the data, it is safe to say that the results of several trials, involving millions of women in the United States and in Europe, do not show that HRT is protective against CVD.

For patients, and even for many clinicians, such results are confusing and even contradictory at times. There may be several possible reasons that could account for this result. A woman's menstrual cycle is probably the most complex biological event in the human body. There are numerous interacting hormones that ebb and flow during the menstrual cycle and over a lifetime. These hormone levels change with age, emotional states, and pregnancy. Besides the many hormones involved, it is likely that there may be other yet undiscovered substances that may play a role in the menstrual cycle. During pregnancy there are still other hormones that come into complex interplay with existing hormones. The replacement of such a complex system cannot be achieved with one simple daily dose of a single hormone or a combination of hormones.

The most popular estrogen used for HRT is Premarin made from mares' urine. Estrone is the major hormone in Premarin, along with equilin and equilenin. Estrone, incidentally, is the kind of estrogen found in postmenopausal women. It is not at all clear that these processed equine hormonal substances mimic in any way what goes on normally in a woman's body. For decades Premarin has been prescribed to postmenopausal women with the naive idea that somehow this substitute estrogen will protect against CVD, osteoporosis, and other symptoms. Though Premarin may alleviate hot flashes and emotional liability in women going through menopause, the more complex issue of the prevention of CVD is not so easily resolved. Given these considerations, it is not surprising that the results of the HRT trials are not definitive.

The American Heart Association (AHA) states, "There is neither a compelling reason to initiate ERT/HRT in a woman for the sole purpose of primary CHD prevention nor a compelling reason to discontinue it if she is doing well with therapy."

The AHA guidance after reviewing the trials reads as follows, "These data suggest no overall cardiovascular benefit and a possible early increased risk of CVD events when HRT is initiated in women with documented atherosclerosis."

Basically, HRT does not seem to have a role in either primary or secondary prevention of heart disease. In fact, estrogen and progestin therapy increases a woman's risk for heart attacks, stroke, blood clots, and breast cancer. Endometrial cancer is also a risk during HRT. Estrogen/progestin also seems to increase the risk of dementia. If a woman needs HRT for hot flashes or other menopausal symptoms, she and her doctor should make a joint decision on its use on a short-term basis after a careful discussion of its risks and benefits.

SUMMARY OF STUDIES RELATED TO THIS CHAPTER

1. Center for Disease Control and Prevention (CDC) guidelines for hypertension, high cholesterol and obesity, physical activity, smoking, and diet: http://www.cdc.gov/heartdisease/guidelines_recommendations.htm
2. CDC guidelines for stroke prevention: http://www.cdc.gov/stroke/guidelines_recommendations.htm
3. American Heart Association primary prevention guidelines: http://circ.ahajournals.org/content/97/18/1876.full
4. Recommendations for secondary prevention of cardiovascular diseases: http://circ.ahajournals.org/content/113/19/2363.full
5. Menopausal hormone replacement therapy: http://www.nih.gov/PHTidex.htm

13

Future Trends in Heart Disease

Any sufficiently advanced technology is indistinguishable from magic.

— Arthur C. Clarke's Third Law

Case Study

Alexis, a 26-year-old PhD graduate student in cell biology, was running up a flight of stairs rushing to class at noon when she felt faint and almost passed out. She sat down for a few minutes and felt better. As she had skipped breakfast that morning, she thought her faintness was due to low blood sugar. When she was 13, her father was found dead on a country road near their home in Connecticut where he had gone jogging. There was no sign of trauma to suggest a car had hit him. He was a successful stockbroker, had no known heart disease, and was thought to be in perfect health. At autopsy, he was found to have hypertrophic cardiomyopathy (HCM). Alexis did not know much about the disease, but recollected reading that HCM may be inherited and fainting spells may precede sudden death. She was training for the Boston Marathon, but she immediately stopped her daily running and competing in 10-kilometer races. The dizzy spell did not recur, but after four months she thought it best to consult a cardiologist who was an expert in HCM.

According to her cardiologist, the physical examination was completely normal. Despite no evidence of abnormalities on cardiac testing, which included an electrocardiogram (EKG), a Holter monitor, an echocardiogram, and a stress test, she was told she needed a myocardial biopsy. This seemed a rather frightening thought, and she declined this option. Genetic testing was not done. Though her cardiologist was also a woman, there was poor communication between them, so she sought another opinion.

Alexis appeared very worried about her condition during her visit to my clinic. She was a very fit and lean blonde, five feet and six inches in height, and seemed the very picture of health. Her arm span was normal and her fingers were not long and tapering, suggesting she did not have evidence for Marfan syndrome. Her blood pressure was 100/70 millimeters of mercury and the heart rate was 60 per minute. The heart sounds were normal and no murmurs were heard. The rest of the examination was, likewise, completely normal.

The resting 12-lead EKG and a 48-hour Holter monitor recording did not show any important rhythm disturbances. She was able to run 16 minutes on a treadmill stress test, which was normal for her age. There were no rhythm abnormalities while running at full speed and nor were there any changes of ischemia. Two-dimensional echocardiography was normal, showing none of the heart muscle thickening changes of HCM from which her father died. The valvular structures were within normal limits.

Much to her relief, I told her that she did not need a myocardial biopsy. A cardiac MRI was recommended, as this study would further confirm that she did not have changes of HCM. As she declined genetic testing, I suggested careful follow-up consisting of regular checkups with electrocardiograms and echocardiograms in six months and then yearly after that, to determine if there was a late manifestation of HCM. I also suggested she follow a normal exercise program in the interim with a six-month follow-up. For the present she was permitted to run three miles a day, but not engage in long competitive races. She wore a portable EKG monitor while running to determine if there were any arrhythmias while running. She would also wore an EKG monitor continuously for a month that would record her heart rhythm in case she got any more dizzy spells. There were no arrhythmias detected and she is free of symptoms after 2 years of follow-up.

The scientific model that developed in the modern era beginning in the 16th century consisted primarily of physician-anatomists examining internal organs at autopsy, searching for a disease process as the cause of death. Abnormal autopsy findings drew the attention of clinicians who attempted to diagnose the disease in life before the patient died. In cases such as rupture of an internal organ or a large tumor, the cause of death could be deduced. However, in the majority of cases, the causes of death could not be determined, as gross anatomy often did not reveal the physiological process leading to death. Moreover, there were no treatments for most conditions other than surgical excision of tumors, removal of blockages in intestines, or the extraction of bladder stones. Medicines rarely worked, except for opium for pain, quinine for fevers, and digitalis for dropsy. These treatments were empirical and none was really curative as the actual causes of the diseases were unknown. Trial and error was the basic "scientific method" of the time!

The physical sciences began their ascent in the 16th century, especially in the fields of astronomy, physics, chemistry, and geology. William Harvey published *De Motu Coris* in 1628, but advances in the biological sciences progressed little thereafter and real advances did not occur until the 19th century. Based on the bedrock of the physical sciences, biological scientists and engineers invented devices that made it possible to understand how the body functioned. The microscope made it possible to discover the germ theory of infectious diseases, pioneered by Louis Pasteur and Robert Koch. The invention of the EKG in the early 20th century eventually uncovered the cause of sudden cardiac death, leading to research that ultimately allowed the complete reversal of this fatal arrhythmia by defibrillation by the mid-century.

The 20th century saw unprecedented advances and discoveries, as well as large capital investments in scientific research and education. Over 90 percent of all scientists who ever lived are alive today, and they contribute to an ongoing effort of research and development in the science enterprise. Revolutionary ideas, such as airplanes, computers, and defibrillators, seem to have the power to overcome the limitations of nature, leading to Arthur Clarke's observation that advanced technologies have the aura of magical force. In the medical arena, putting someone to sleep and then waking them up with a new heart in the place of the old one sounds like one of Grimms' fairy tales.

The 21st century promises to be the age of biomedical science, particularly in the area of understanding and altering the microscopic composition of cells and their tiny internal components, such as nuclei, chromosomes, and mitochondria. This new era also opens the door to new and innovative treatments targeted at the actual biological processes that cause disease, rather than medications that essentially treat symptoms and effects on end-organs with a hit-or-miss approach. What are the pivotal developments in science that are transforming medical care in the 21st century?

There are *four principal developments* that make the probing and treatment of disease processes possible in the 21st century.

First, cellular and molecular biology and genetics have made major strides in understanding the molecular basis for diseases. Already, specific genes associated with congenital heart disease, high cholesterol, and certain other types of cardiovascular disease have been identified, making prediction of such diseases possible. Genetic manipulation is thus possible to cure various diseases.

Understanding the genetic basis for diseases also makes the targeted use of drug therapy for specific diseases possible. This means that trial and error in treatment of cardiovascular disease will be replaced by selectively using drugs that will benefit the patient. Though this process will probably take decades to be completed, specific drugs that are released over a period of time from biological cells implanted within the body will be developed to treat cancer, rhythm disturbances, and infections.

Second, the development of new high-technology devices, like the new metallic, nonmetallic, and biosynthetic materials, makes it possible to replace parts of the cardiovascular system. The body has powerful reactions to foreign materials introduced into the body, even if they are biological in nature. The challenge to material scientists is to produce materials that will stay within the body and substitute for a biological function without provoking serious side effects, and without being damaged or destroyed. Such materials either replace worn-out parts, such as a diseased aorta, or replace an entire organ, such as the heart. Such high-technology approaches are often coupled with robotic surgery to allow operations through "keyholes" in the body. Such surgery is minimally invasive and increases accuracy while operating on the heart and other organs, reducing trauma to the body and decreasing a patient's hospital stay.

Third, miniaturization of electrical circuits and batteries makes it possible to create small devices that can be implanted to substitute for damaged or diseased parts of the body. The best examples to date are the implantable pacemaker and the implantable defibrillator, each of which used to weigh up to a hundred or more pounds.

Fourth, the development of powerful computers with massive computing power allows the collection, aggregation, and storage of data sets, making it possible to analyze data that cannot be done by hand or by an individual scientist alone. Subjecting data to analysis using mathematical algorithms allows scientists to understand how complex biological systems interact, discern patterns of disease, and design long-term treatment strategies. Correlations between biological parameters and psychosocial variables can be discerned by multivariate analyses in large population groups that cannot be done by human brain alone. The testing of possible treatment strategies and interventions in test populations is possible in order to calculate outcomes in order to validate such treatments statistically. Side effects and unintended consequences of treatment can also be tracked for safety to detect therapeutic mishaps early when large numbers of subjects are being treated with a new drug.

These developments have largely occurred in the last 50 years, and they will be dealt with selectively as they apply to several different conditions in the treatment of heart disease.

GENOMICS AND GENETICS

The *genome* is the genetic structure of a cell. *Genomics* is the study of genes, their composition, and the sequencing and alteration of genes by various laboratory techniques. *Genetics* is the study of heredity in plants and animals. Clinical genetics is the study of how families inherit certain biological characteristics. The study of genetically transmitted disease is one of the most promising new areas in terms of treating heart disease. It makes it possible to diagnose a disease using genetic testing and then target the disease through *genomic medicine*. This is an exciting possibility and early experimental methods are being tried.

Alexis thought she might have inherited hypertrophic cardiomyopathy (HCM) from her father, who died relatively young. In the United States, HCM is the most common inherited form of heart disease. When an athlete collapses and dies on the basketball court or football field, this disease is often the first disease suspected. Hypertrophic cardiomyopathy was recognized only about 50 years ago, and its genetic basis was discovered more recently. A gene for HCM is inherited as an *autosomal dominant* gene from one parent. This condition leads to both anatomical abnormalities in heart muscle as well as electrical disorders that can lead to sudden death. Alexis's condition poses one of the dilemmas in modern medicine, which is what should be done in the case of inherited genetic disease. Should she be benched and forbidden to exercise? Should she have children? How should she be treated? These are all open questions because we still lack sufficient data to provide precise answers.

Sometimes one parent has a defective, but dominant gene, or both parents have recessive genes that can be passed on to offspring. When present alone or together, such dominant genes can cause a disease such as familial hypercholesterolemia, as in the case of Stormie Jones in the previous chapter. In other cases, mutations in genes can cause the disease to spring up spontaneously. Genetic defects also occur when deletion of certain genes or part of a chromosome occurs, or if an extra chromosome is inherited. The latter occurs in Down syndrome, when three copies of chromosome 21 exist in the same cell.

There are many heart diseases that are genetically based, such as Turner and Williams syndromes. In Turner syndrome, one sex chromosome is missing so genetically the person is female, but has nonworking ovaries and therefore cannot have children and pass this defect on. Turner syndrome females may also have atrial septal defect, aortic stenosis, or coarctation of the aorta. In Williams syndrome, the child is extremely friendly and cheerful, will go off with practically anyone as he or she has a "cocktail party" kind of personality, and will often fail to discriminate situations of danger. This syndrome affects 1 in 10,000 people worldwide, and it is known to occur equally in both males and females. An estimated 20,000 to 30,000 people in the United States have this condition. Cardiovascular defects associated with this condition include coarctation of the aorta and pulmonary artery narrowing.

Marfan syndrome is another genetic disorder and involves connective tissue that can be inherited as a dominant trait. The gene FBN1 controls a connective tissue protein called *fibrillin-1*. People with Marfan syndrome are typically tall with long limbs and long, tapering fingers. With this condition, the elastic and connective tissue that holds heart valves and the three layers of the aorta breaks down over many years. This results in mitral and aortic valve leakage and a disruption of the architecture of the aorta. Expansion of the valve ring leads to aortic or mitral valve insufficiency, causing leakage of blood.

Dilation of the aorta and tearing in the middle layer in the wall of the aorta along its length result in a condition called dissection. The dissection of the ascending aorta as it comes off the left ventricle can involve the coronary arteries and cause chest pain. This condition, which can lead to bleeding into the wall of the aorta, is followed by death. As alluded to earlier, this is how Jonathan Larson, the musician and composer of the rock musical *Rent*, died. He was found dead in his apartment the day before his musical opened in New York City. Sadly, the diagnosis was missed earlier in the day in two emergency rooms where he was seen for chest pains. Screening techniques in the future for diseases such as for Marfan syndrome will identify the disease state, and improved surveillance for possible victims will allow preventive strategies to be put in place.

Other genetic anomalies can lead to electrical abnormalities in the heart that result in sudden death in infants or young adults. These include congenital long QT interval syndrome and Brugada syndrome. The former can be inherited as an autosomal dominant or as a recessive gene, while the Brugada syndrome is inherited as a dominant gene.

Propensity for myocardial infarction is also genetically based. A fairly common condition is familial hypercholesterolemia that causes high levels of "bad" cholesterol (LDL cholesterol) beginning at birth. One out of 500 people in the United States inherits this condition, as we have discussed earlier.

While more and more new genetic diseases are discovered, many are not treatable because there has been little clinical experience with them. Genetic defects generally cannot presently be corrected, but the resulting symptoms can often be treated. Treatments have to be fashioned by trial and error, and doctors have to make sure that the cure is not worse than the disease.

In the future, genetic defects can be cured with gene replacement therapy, and attempts are now being done experimentally. The method is ingenious and consists of inserting the needed gene into a virus. Viruses are made up of deoxyribonucleic acid (DNA) or ribonucleic acid (RNA) and can only replicate inside a cell. The virus used as the vector is usually an *adenovirus*. The virus carrying the needed DNA infects cells in the host's body. The cell then goes on to manufacture the missing protein, thus correcting the deficiency. Unfortunately, if the genetic defect, such as an atrial or ventricular septal defect, is already established in the heart anatomically at birth, this type of treatment is not likely to be of help.

STEM CELLS AND HEART REPAIR

In 2006, Shinya Yamanaka, a Japanese physician and stem cell researcher, turned adult mouse fibroblasts into adult stem cells called *induced pluripotent stem cells* (iPSC). The following year, he and his colleagues turned human fibroblasts into iPSC as well. The reprogramming of adult fibroblasts into precursors of other cells (e.g., heart, kidney, or liver cells) holds promise, though it should be cautioned that such cells might also have similarity to cancer cells. The 2012 Nobel Prize in Physiology or Medicine was awarded to Yamanaka and John Gurdon for their work that mature cells can be reprogrammed to become pluripotent.

After a myocardial infarction, or in cardiomyopathy, there is dead scar tissue that does not contract; and pumping action of the ventricle is reduced. Deepak Srivastava, a cardiologist at the Gladstone Institute affiliated with the University of California in San Francisco, has applied Yamanaka's technique in pigs to convert scar or connective tissue cells to muscle by manipulating native cells into contractile cells. According to him, since about 50 percent of the heart contains fibroblasts, there is a possibility that such cells can be reprogrammed into contractile heart muscle. He is cautiously optimistic that it will be possible to repair the heart muscle by these methods in the future as current stem cell technology is scalable and has the capacity to create billions of muscle cells.

Srivastava says we can expect clinical trials that test delivery of stem cells to the heart during different stages of a myocardial infarction. If done in the early stages of a myocardial infarction, this will start a process of repair before the heart tissue turns to scar tissue, and will allow contractile function to return. Since cardiac pumping action is a determinant of long-term survival after a myocardial infarction, this approach will help increase longevity. Except in the most severe of cases, it may be possible in the distant future that heart valves will be able to be repaired without surgery using a similar method.

The future may well see iPSC cells used to cover an artificial fibrous scaffolding to recreate an entirely new heart made of contractile cells, instead of implanting a metallic mechanical pump like the present iteration of the artificial heart. It is conceivable that an artificially created heart, built on a flexible scaffolding with stem cells with implanted bioprosthetic valves and an implanted pacemaker, could be the first step to manufacturing a heart composed mostly of natural tissue.

Whether stem cell therapy can be used to cure congenital heart disease remains to be seen. It is unlikely that established heart defects could be so treated, as the defect is already present at birth. However, during fetal development, it may be possible to introduce genetic material and reprogram cells to complete a defective process if such a process can be diagnosed in utero. It may thus be possible to use stem cells to grow parts of the septum in atrial and ventricular septal defects in the fetus to correct the hole in the heart.

Futurologists and "singularity" proponents, who are not geneticists or stem cell researchers, have made predictions that three-dimensional printer technology can "print" complete organs in the next 5 to 10 years. Stem cell therapy is not at the stage where such "printing" of organs is anywhere near this time frame. Clifford Tabin, head of genetics at Harvard Medical School, is cautious about making near-term predictions. In his opinion, it may well be 20 years at least before genetic treatments become established therapy for genetic disease. Caution is appropriate, as all treatments, even in the best of hands, have side effects that cannot be predicted ahead of time.

SURGICAL TREATMENTS

Robotic surgery is gaining increasing attention, as described in Chapter 10. Systems such as the da Vinci robot will be used increasingly to guide surgery resulting in less invasive procedures. This system is already used for cardiac, lung, kidney, bladder, prostate, throat, brain, and gynecologic surgery. Its use can be extended to more and more procedures. In due course, it will be routine in isolated regions and on the battlefield for trained assistants to perform surgery using robots under remote visual guidance by specialist surgeons. This development will save lives at an early stage of the disease or injury.

In vascular diseases such as Marfan syndrome, highly invasive surgery is performed to replace the diseased aorta or a major blood vessel. There have been exciting new developments in the field of engineering new bioprosthetic materials for replacement of body parts. Instead of total surgical excision of the aorta and replacement with Gore-Tex grafts, intravascular stent grafts are being now used. These grafts are balloon-expandable and placed inside the existing aorta so that extensive surgical dissection and removal of the native aorta are not necessary. The stent grafts are made of a metallic framework with woven polyester material. Since these grafts were developed only about 10 years ago and have been widely available only since 2005, further development and experiments in biomaterials can be expected to continue. It can be expected that other smaller arteries may be treated in a similar manner. It is also likely that instead of using vein grafts for coronary artery bypass surgery, artificial grafts will be constructed to treat patients with CAD.

In pediatric surgery, a number of investigational procedures are being performed to treat cardiac conditions such as aortic stenosis, pulmonary valve atresia, and hypoplastic left heart syndrome. In most of these cases, the baby will die soon after birth, so treatment should be given before birth. The diagnosis is made by cardiac ultrasound and interventions made as early as the 22nd week of gestation.

James Locke and his cardiology colleagues at the Children's Hospital Medical Center in Boston have pioneered methods to treat these congenital heart conditions. The method consists of using a large-bore needle that penetrates the abdominal wall under ultrasound guidance. The needle penetrates through the uterus, the amniotic sac, and the chest of the fetus to enter the heart, and approaches the defective valve through the wall of the left ventricle. Widening of the valve orifice is done with a dilating instrument. Over 150 cases have been done over the last 10 years, and of these, 90 have been for aortic stenosis. The fetal mortality in the latter cases is low with a remarkable 92 percent survival rate. Such intra-uterine approaches can be expanded to other congenital heart diseases in the future. However, because the number of patients for many congenital diseases is so small, severe limitations in funding in a market economy make rapid development in this field very difficult.

PREDICTION OF MYOCARDIAL INFARCTION

Although clinical characteristics such as age and gender are well-established risk factors for CVD, such features are not sufficient to identify all patients at risk for a heart attack (myocardial infarction). Cardiovascular "biomarkers" are biochemical or genetic tests that allow the assessment of clinical risk for a disease. Sometimes, such markers can not only help with screening, but may also be used for diagnosis, for assessment of prognosis, and for response to treatment. One such simple test that is already widely available is the blood cholesterol level test, which allows diagnosis, risk assessment, and assessment of how well a person is doing on treatment.

However, most such current biomarkers have only approximate predictive value, so that there is a need to identify additional and more precise biomarkers for assessing biological pathways for premature heart disease. *C-reactive protein* and *homocysteine* levels *may* predict the onset of coronary artery disease, but they are not precise enough to have a strong predictive value for when a myocardial infarction or death will occur.

It is likely that in coming years, other biomarkers, based on profiling microcellular components such as DNA, RNA, proteins, and some chemical metabolites in blood or tissues, will help identify propensity for myocardial infarction.

SUDDEN CARDIAC DEATH

The ability to predict the onset of sudden cardiac death (SCD) resulting from ventricular fibrillation (VF) has been an elusive goal, and the search for a reliable predictive test has become the Holy Grail of cardiology. Because it is the number one killer in all Western countries, numerous attempts have already been made to predict SCD. However, there has been little success using these relatively crude tests, such as exercise stress testing, advanced forms of analysis of the electrocardiography, cardiac catheterization, and electrophysiological testing to predict the onset of SCD. The most obvious test is the EKG, which can be done in a doctor's office. Attempts at fast Fourier transformation analysis of signal-averaged EKGs have been used to identify patients who are at risk for cardiac arrest. With the exception of long QT interval syndrome, so far, it is not possible for such tests to predict SCD with any accuracy. Still, as described earlier, genetic testing for conditions such as Brugada syndrome provides a diagnosis in 20 percent of cases.

The ideal will be to find a relatively inexpensive and easily done test to identify future victims. Further development of such methods will provide an early indicator of potential premature death. It is likely that a combination of parameters will be used to determine if someone will die suddenly from cardiac arrest in the future. Such a test will include electrophysiological mapping of the heart along with a three-dimensional gene expression cardiac map of the heart. Such a genomic map will be similar to that developed for the brain by the Allen Institute for Brain Science. Such a genomic map of the heart could be useful for predicting sudden cardiac death in the future.

It will be possible to genetically reprogram cells to insert genetic material to correct deleted genes for a variety of diseases that result in SCD. If this type of treatment can be performed and the electrophysiological abnormalities corrected, it will save countless lives. This process will prevent sudden death without the need to insert an implantable defibrillator to protect the person when cardiac arrest occurs. Corrective treatments of this type address the underlying causes of cardiac arrest, rather than treating it once it has occurred.

DRUG DEVELOPMENT

The majority of heart diseases are treated with drugs and not by surgery. Drugs are the mainstay of many heart conditions. Therefore, new drugs are under development for conditions such as angina, high cholesterol, arrhythmias, congestive heart failure, and high blood pressure. New drugs are necessary because many existing drugs have serious toxic effects, including death, as they interfere directly with cardiac function. If a patient experiences a side effect, an alternate drug has to be used.

Drugs given orally or by injection are distributed all over the body—to more or less all organs. Only a small portion of the drug reaches the heart. So, it is preferable to have drugs treat only the organ that is affected. Targeted drug delivery is a method of delivering the curative agent specifically only to the organ that is affected by a disease process. The drug is delivered to the organ by a substance called a liposome, or by a polymer that attaches only to that organ so that generalized distribution of the drug throughout the body is avoided. Clearly, this method will avoid or reduce side effects of the drug on other organs.

There is also the developing field of *nanotechnology*. In this branch of science, matter is manipulated on an atomic or molecular level. In DNA nanotechnology, artificial DNA is created for the specific purpose of treating abnormal cells. Researchers have created a *biologically programmable computing machine* composed of enzymes and DNA instead of silicon chips. There is reason to speculate that such biological DNA-based logic circuits can be programmed to release drugs within cells in response to certain types of disease states such as cancer. If the heart cells produce abnormal electrical stimuli or have abnormalities in contraction, it is possible that such nanotechnology tools can be used to repair and correct the abnormalities.

At present, drugs are tested directly on patients, and their effects determined over time to assess effectiveness. In the future, it is likely that drugs will be tested on clusters of a patient's cells. Genomic sequencing has gotten simpler and drugs may be specifically designed to affect genetic targets. As described earlier, *induced pluripotent stem cells* (iPSC) can be created from fibroblast cells. Such cells can be used for testing of drug effectiveness by acting as a surrogate phenotypic marker. The activity and response of a large cluster of such cells may provide an indication whether the drug will be effective. We are still a long way away in terms of applying such targeted treatment with "intelligent drugs." If this approach is successful, the use of invasive cardiac procedures and surgery can be reduced.

LONGEVITY RESEARCH

The quest for immortality has also been the Holy Grail of alchemists, scientists, New Age enthusiasts, and modern-day investigators, such as Aubrey de Gray and Ray Kurzweil. Texts such as the Bible, as well as tracts in Hinduism, Buddhism, Zoroastrianism, and the Epic of Gilgamesh, all speak to immortality in the afterlife of the soul.

Extension of life span is realistic in the modern era. In the Neolithic age, life span was estimated to be 20 years, and in pre-Columbian America it was about 25–35 years. In 1900, life expectancy was 47 years, and by 2000, it was 78 years in Western Europe and North America—a remarkable increase of 66 percent. The initial increase in longevity seen in the early 20th century was due to better sanitation, safe water supply, better housing, and safer childbirth due to control of sepsis.

After 1940, the role of antibiotics, better surgical techniques, and safer anesthesia to treat acute conditions and major injuries played a role in increasing longevity. From the 1960s on, the introduction of beta-adrenergic blocking agents, aspirin, ACE inhibitors, statins to control cholesterol level, pacemakers, and CPR to reverse cardiac arrest all played a role in prolonging life. Heart transplants and surgery for congenital heart and coronary artery disease played an important, but smaller, role in increasing longevity.

Deaths from heart disease declined 69 percent from 1950 to 2006, with a marked change occurring after 1968. This decline coincides with the progressive and widespread use of beta-blocker drugs, aspirin, ACE inhibitors, and statins. Control of risk factors such as smoking and diabetes and better dietary habits also contributed to the decline in coronary heart disease mortality. Recently, vitamin supplements, coenzyme Q10, acai berry, pomegranate and mangosteen juice, antioxidants, and other supplements have been promoted as having healthful effects on the heart and on life in general. While antioxidants have a role in maintaining health, there is no evidence at present that such supplements have a therapeutic role, and they have no proven role in prolonging life. However, it is realistic to imagine that genuine and proven biochemically active agents will be found that can be shown to delay aging and prolong life.

SUMMARY

None of the "miracles" of modern medicine would have been possible without the talents of dedicated scientists and biomedical engineers. The wizardry of biomedical engineering combined with the skills of basic scientists, cardiologists, and surgeons have already wrought major changes in the treatment of diseases of the heart.

Advances in genetics, cellular biology, nanobiotechnology, pharmacology, materials science, digital technology, electronics, and optics will accelerate both diagnosis and therapy of heart disease. Advanced imaging technologies and miniaturization allow for the direct and indirect visualization of the interior of blood vessels and cardiac structures, allowing for more accurate diagnoses to be made. These methods will also allow further advances in robotic surgery as imaging technologies are further refined. Stem cell and gene therapy will repair damaged tissue and defective chromosomes. Rehabilitation from surgery and following myocardial infarction will change dramatically by the use of new less invasive methods that allow for speedy recovery.

While it is extremely difficult to accurately predict the future of medicine, these advances in conceptual thinking, innovation, and new technology will change how heart disease is diagnosed and treated.

Time Line

that the heart, rather than the brain, was the source of human wisdom, emotions, memory, the soul, and personality itself. It was through the heart that God spoke, giving ancient Egyptians knowledge of God and God's will. For this reason, it was considered the most important of the body's organs.

130–200 CE   Galen, the great Greek physician, saw the brain as the center of reason, the heart as the seat of emotion, and the liver as the seat of passion. He presents the idea of two kinds of blood—"nutritive" blood made by the liver and "vital" blood made by the heart and pumped through arteries. The heart remains the source of heat, and the blood cools as it circulates. He assumes that blood traverses the ventricular septum, from one side of the heart to the other, through tiny pores. The lungs were believed to have a fanning and cooling function on the heart.

1213–1288   Ibn al-Nafis, an Arab physician, is the first person to accurately describe pulmonary circulation. He challenges the long-held view of the Galen school that blood can pass through the cardiac interventricular septum though microscopic pores. He believed that blood passed through the lungs to reach the heart. This required connection, at some level, between the pulmonary artery and vein.

1452–1519   Leonardo da Vinci sketches detailed and accurate drawings of the heart based on dissections. He does not publish these diagrams.

1460–1530   Jacopo Berengario da Carpi accurately describes the chambers of the heart.

1628   William Harvey publishes *Exercitatio Anatomica de Motu Cordis et Sanguinis in Animalibus* (An Anatomical Exercise on the Motion of the Heart and Blood in Living Beings), which captures the mechanical workings of the heart. He does the first detailed experiments on animals showing that the heart has interlocking circulatory systems with different functions, establishing the scientific basis for quantitative thinking in biology.

1733   Stephen Hales publishes *Haemastaticks*. He was the first to measure blood pressure directly by inserting a glass tube into the carotid artery in the neck of a horse.

1775	Peder Christian Abildgaard (1740–1801) shocks electrocuted chickens back to life using electric discharges from Leyden jars.
1816	René Théophile Hyacinthe Laënnec (1781–1826) invents the stethoscope, allegedly after witnessing children playing near the Louvre, listening to the ends of long pieces of timber that transmitted the sounds of pin scratches. He mills a hollow wooden cylinder that he uses to listen to the chest sounds of his patients. Laënnec referred to his instrument as the stethoscope.
1857	Étienne-Jules Marey (1830–1904) invents the wrist sphygmograph to measure blood pressure. Robert Ellis Dudgeon (1820–1904) improves upon Dr. Marey's model in 1881. He creates an instrument that captures the pulse at the wrist, causing a metal strip to move a stylus, and thus transmitting the record of the pulse onto smoked paper on a rotating drum. Siegfried von Basch (1837–1905) from Vienna also develops a similar instrument, the sphygmomanometer, a portable noninvasive instrument for measuring blood pressure in 1881. The Italian internist and pediatrician Scipione Riva Rocci (1863–1937) invents a sphygmomanometer to measure blood pressure in 1896 with an inflatable arm cuff (to compress the brachial artery in the arm).
1860–1880s	Michael Foster (1836–1907) and Carl Ludwig (1816–1895) posit that the heart is an electromechanical organ. The laboratories of both Foster and Ludwig established that though the heart and the brain were closely linked, the heart could also beat independently of the nervous system. Scientists at both laboratories also worked on the electrical system of the heart. They show that this internal wiring, called the *conduction system*, is the component that keeps the heart beating rhythmically.
1873	In France, Gabriel Lippmann (1845–1921) invents the capillary electrometer that is used to record the first electrocardiogram.
1876	Étienne-Jules Marey records the first electrocardiogram (EKG) in Paris using a mercury capillary electrometer. A column of mercury in the glass capillary moved up and down when it detected a tiny flow of electrical current passing

through it. By using this device in London in 1887, Augustus Waller (1856–1922) indirectly records the electrical activity of the human heart by using electrodes attached to the surface of the body.

1889   John MacWilliam (1857–1937), a Scottish physician and physiologist, proposes that ventricular fibrillation is the heartbeat rhythm primarily responsible for sudden death in humans. He bases this theory on the newly emerging field of evolutionary biology. Charles Darwin had published his *Origin of Species* in 1858; MacWilliam saw a phylogenetic similarity between the electrical behavior of hearts progressing from fish to frog to man. His theory was eventually proven in the late 20th century when doctors became aware that heart attack deaths were most often due to ventricular fibrillation.

1899   Jean Louis Prevost and Frederic Battelli in Geneva, Switzerland, show that small currents cause ventricular fibrillation and large currents terminate it.

1903   Willem Einthoven (1860–1927) develops the EKG into a practical clinical diagnostic tool. He uses multiple electrical leads positioned on different parts of the body to triangulate the electrical activity of the heart and record EKGs. By looking at the heart from different angles he was able to create a sort of electrical map of the heart. Einthoven also gave the names to the waves of the EKG, following the Descartes convention for naming points on mathematical diagrams: P, Q, R, S, and T.

1912   James Herrick (1861–1954) is the first to suggest that a "heart attack" (myocardial infarction) was due to coronary thrombosis. He suggests that the coronary arteries feeding the heart with blood and oxygen become clogged with clots, thus causing a heart attack.

1913   George Ralph Mines (1886–1914) discovers one of the keystone concepts of cardiac electrophysiology known as the *vulnerable period* of the heart. During a very brief period in the cardiac cycle, an external stimulus, such as an electrical pulse or a blow to the heart, can trigger ventricular fibrillation and cause cardiac arrest and sudden death.

1915	A pioneering group of physicians and social workers form the first Association for the Prevention and Relief of Heart Disease in New York City.
1924	Willem Einthoven wins the Nobel Prize in Medicine for producing a clinically useful EKG device.
1924	Recognizing the need for a national organization to share research findings and promote further study, six cardiologists representing several groups found the American Heart Association. The mission of the American Heart Association was to disseminate knowledge of cardiovascular disease by enlisting help from thousands of physicians and scientists and to engage the public in improving cardiac health.
1929	Werner Forssmann (1904–1979) passes a urinary catheter into his own heart via a vein after anesthetizing his own arm. He then walks down a flight of stairs to the radiology department and takes an X-ray of his heart, which shows that the catheter is located in the right atrium.
1932	Albert Hyman (with his brother Charles) performs cardiac pacing and calls the device an *artificial pacemaker*.
1937	John Heysham Gibbon (1903–1973) invents the heart-lung bypass machine, which is the first to provide artificial circulation. He later performs the first open heart surgery.
1940s	William Bennett Kouwenhoven (1886–1975), an engineer at the Physics Laboratory at Johns Hopkins University in Baltimore, and his colleagues find that electrical currents, while causing ventricular fibrillation, could be used to reverse it as well. They also discover the basis for cardiopulmonary resuscitation.
1947	Claude Beck (1994–1971), a surgeon, uses the defibrillator on a human for the first time in Cleveland, Ohio.
1948	President Harry S. Truman signs the National Heart Act, creating and establishing the National Heart Institute. The National Heart, Lung and Blood Institute starts the Framingham Heart Study in Massachusetts.
1952	Charles Hufnagel (1916–1989) is the first surgeon to place an artificial valve in the aorta of a 30-year-old woman. This

is later repeated by Dwight Harken in 1960, and Albert Starr and M. E. Edwards in 1961.

1955   Paul Zoll (1911–1999), in Boston, defibrillates a human through an intact chest using an AC defibrillator.

1956   André F. Cournand, Werner Forssmann, and Dickinson W. Richards share the Nobel Prize "on their discoveries concerning heart catheterization and pathological changes in the circulatory system."

1957   Earl Bakken (b. 1924) invents the first practical external pacemaker box in his garage in Minneapolis, Minnesota.

1958   First pacemaker implantation done at the Karolinska Institute, Stockholm, Sweden, on Arne Larsson.

1960   F. Mason Sones Jr. (1918–1985), a pediatric cardiologist at the Cleveland Clinic in Ohio, accidentally injects opaque radiographic dye into the coronary artery of a patient and is able to visualize the coronary arteries. He goes on to combine cardiac catheterization with coronary angiography and high-speed X-ray cinematography to visualize the coronary arteries. Using this procedure it is possible to see blockages in the coronary arteries.

1960s   Michael DeBakey (1908–2008) and David Sabiston (1924–2009) separately perform what is known today as coronary artery bypass surgery (CABG).

1963   Bernard Lown introduces cardioversion using direct current to revert stable cardiac arrhythmias by adding a timing device to defibrillators to avoid causing ventricular fibrillation.

1965   Frank Pantridge in Belfast, Ireland, starts mobile coronary care unit for early response to myocardial infarction and cardiac arrest using small portable defibrillators.

1967   Christiaan Barnard (1922–2001), a surgeon in South Africa, transplants the first human heart from Denise Darvall into Louis Washkansky, who lives for 18 days, only to die from pneumonia.

1967   Adrian Kantrowitz (1918–2008) performs the first human heart transplant in the United States, by transplanting a heart from a brain-dead baby to another baby. The baby with the newly transplanted heart survives only six hours.

1969   Domingo Liotta (b. 1924) and Denton Cooley (b. 1920) implant the first artificial heart.

1976   Akira Endo in Japan discovers and isolates a statin drug from the fungus *Aspergillus terre* that is used to lower blood cholesterol.

1977   Andreas Gruentzig (1939–1985), a German radiologist, is the first to perform balloon angioplasty. He inserts a catheter with an inflatable balloon into a coronary artery. Then, by applying hydrostatic pressure to inflate the balloon, he squishes plaque in a coronary artery to open the artery up and increase blood flow. This procedure is called interventional cardiology or angioplasty.

1980   Morton Mower and Michel Mirowski (1924–1990) develop an implantable defibrillator. The first implantation of the device will take place that year at Johns Hopkins Hospital in Baltimore, Maryland.

1980s   Coronary stents are implanted in coronary arteries opened by angioplasty by a variety of investigators, reducing restenosis by keeping the artery open. Drug-eluting stents followed in the 1990s.

1981   Beta-adrenergic blocking drugs are shown to decrease mortality after myocardial infarction in European and American studies.

1985   Michael S. Brown (b. 1941) and Joseph L. Goldstein (b. 1940) from Dallas, Texas, share the Nobel Prize for showing how cholesterol is made and regulated in the liver.

2003   The Human Genome Project is completed, mapping 25,000 genes in humans, opening the way to cure genetically based cardiovascular and other diseases such as familial hypercholesterolemia as well as Marfan, Turner, Down, and other syndromes.

2007   Shinya Yamanaka (b. 1962) from Japan turns human fibroblasts into adult stem cells, opening the way for the possible repair of damaged heart muscles using stem cell therapy.

Glossary

Ablation: The electrical or surgical removal or destruction of cardiac tissue or conduction pathways in the heart involved in arrhythmias.

Algorithm: A set of rules, guidelines, or procedures for clinical care. Computer algorithms are rules programmed into a pacemaker or defibrillator designed for reacting to and solving specific problems.

Anastomosis: The surgical joining of two hollow organs or tubes, such as blood vessels or intestines.

Aneurysm: A bulging or dilation of part of a blood vessel due to weakening of the wall.

Angina: A sensation in the chest that occurs often with exertion, in the cold, or with emotional stress that is due to lack of blood flow to heart muscle.

Angiography: The radiographic study of blood vessels by the injection of dye into the vessel (see catheterization).

Angioplasty: The opening of a narrowed artery using a balloon catheter inflated with saline to crush plaque to improve blood flow.

Anticoagulant: A medicine that prevents blood from clotting.

Anti-tachycardia pacing: Short, rapid bursts of pacing pulses delivered by an implantable cardioverter-defibrillator (ICD) and used to terminate an arrhythmia in the atria or ventricles.

Arrest (cardiac): Cessation of the heart's normal rhythmic electrical and/or mechanical activity, which causes loss of pulse and blood pressure.

Arrhythmia: A heart rhythm that falls outside the accepted normal range for rate and regularity and form of the P wave and/or QRS complex.

Arterioles: Small blood vessels that are intermediate in size between arteries and capillaries.

Arteriosclerosis: A chronic disease that causes thickening, hardening, and loss of elasticity of the arterial walls resulting in impaired blood circulation. It develops with aging, hypertension, and diabetes.

Asystole: Complete stoppage of all electrical activity of the heart.

Atheroma: Collection of fatty plaque inside a blood vessel adhering to the wall; similar to *plaque*.

Atherosclerosis: A form of arteriosclerosis that is caused by a buildup of cholesterol, calcium, and plaque in the inner lining of an artery.

Atrial fibrillation (AF): Disorganized and chaotic heart rhythm in the atria with wormlike movement, usually occurring about 300 to 500 times a minute.

Atrial flutter: Organized regular atrial rhythm occurring about 300 times a minute.

Atrial tachycardia: A rapid heart rate that starts in the atria, usually applied to regular rhythms, and often denotes rhythms other than atrial fibrillation and flutter. This rhythm is also called paroxysmal atrial tachycardia (PAT).

Atrioventricular (AV) node: A collection of specialized electrically active cells that are part of the normal conduction pathway between the atria and the ventricles. It has a gating function between the atria to the ventricles of the heart; often also referred to as the *junction*.

Atrium: The heart is divided into four chambers. Each of the two upper chambers is called an *atrium*. *Atria* is the plural form.

Bradyarrhythmia: Any slow rhythm below the rate of 60 beats per minute.

Bradycardia: A heart rate that is under 60 beats per minute and often refers specifically to sinus rhythm.

Bruit: A sound heard over a blood vessel due to flow of blood through a narrowing in the artery or vein.

Capillaries: These are the smallest vessels that bridge arteries and veins and deliver oxygen and nutrients to body tissues.

Cardiac arrest: Failure of the heart to pump enough blood through the body. If left untreated, it results in sudden death.

Cardiomyopathy: Weakening and damage of the heart muscle caused by a disease process resulting in reduced pumping action.

Cardioversion: Termination of an atrial or ventricular tachyarrhythmia by the delivery of DC current that is synchronized to the R wave of the EKG.

Catheterization: The procedure of inserting a hollow tube into a blood vessel and threading the tube to the heart to measure blood pressure, or to inject dye in order to study the anatomy and physiology of the heart and its arteries.

Computer-assisted tomography (CAT or CT scan): Examination of a body part using X-rays and computer processing to recreate two- or three-dimensional images.

Congenital: A condition or disease existing at birth.

Coronary artery: One of two arteries that arise from the aorta (or one of their lesser branches) that supplies blood to the heart muscle.

Coronary artery bypass grafting (CABG): Surgery in which a blood vessel is grafted to the coronary artery to bypass the blocked section of a coronary artery to improve blood supply to the heart.

Cyanosis: The blue color of the skin, lips, and nails caused by venous blood when it is low in oxygen. This condition is seen in congenital heart disease.

Defibrillation: Termination of ventricular fibrillation by unsynchronized direct current delivered to the heart through the chest or through electrodes placed within the heart.

Diastole: The relaxation phase of the heart following contraction of the heart muscle.

Diuretic: A medicine that acts on the kidney to remove water from the body.

Dual-chamber pacemaker: A pacemaker with two leads (one in the atrium and one in the ventricle) to allow pacing and/or sensing in both chambers of the heart to artificially restore the natural contraction sequence of the heart.

Echocardiography: The use of ultrasound to measure and record the size, motion, and composition of various cardiac structures in the diagnosis of heart disease.

Edema: Swelling of a body part from the abnormal accumulation of fluid (spelled *oedema* in British English).

Effusion: A collection of fluid in a body cavity.

Ejection fraction: A measure of the output of blood from the heart with each heartbeat; it is calculated by dividing stroke volume by end-diastolic volume.

Electrocardiogram (ECG or EKG): A printout from an electrocardiography machine used to measure and record the electrical activity of the heart.

Electrode: An insulated wire or a catheter that conducts electricity and is used to record electrical activity from the heart, or deliver an electric charge to the heart. It is also called a *lead* (leed).

Electromagnetic interference/pulse (EMI or EMP): Equipment and appliances that use magnets and electricity have electromagnetic fields around them. If these fields are strong, they may interfere with the operation of an implantable pacemaker or defibrillator, causing them to malfunction.

Electrophysiology (EP) study: The use of programmed electrical stimulation to assess the electrical activity of the heart in order to diagnose arrhythmias.

Embolus: A clot that travels from the heart or a blood vessel to another part of the circulation and lodges at a remote location. The process is called *embolization* (see thrombus).

Endocardium: The thin innermost lining that covers the inside of the heart.

Endotracheal tube: A tube inserted into the trachea (windpipe) to provide a passageway for air to enter the lungs and to allow ventilation.

Epicardium: The thin layer that covers the outside of the heart.

Fibrillation: A chaotic and unsynchronized worm-like movement of the myocardium during which no effective pumping occurs. Fibrillation can occur in both the atria and the ventricles.

Heart attack: A lay term that refers to any cardiac event such as severe chest pain or cardiac arrest. It often refers to myocardial infarction or to cardiac arrest, but it is not specific enough to describe the exact cause or the exact medical diagnosis.

Heart block: A condition in which electrical impulses are not conducted normally from the atria to the ventricles. It is caused by damage or disease processes within the cardiac conduction system. This is not a physical or mechanical "blockage," but rather an electrical impediment to the flow of an electrical impulse within the heart.

Hemodynamics: The forces involved in circulating blood through the cardiovascular system. Also used to refer collectively to the combination of measurements of heart rate, blood pressure, contractility, cardiac output, and other physical measurements of heart function that can be expressed as mathematical equations.

Holter monitoring: A technique for the continuous recording of electrocardiographic signals on tape or digitally, usually over 24–48 hours, to detect and diagnose ECG changes; also called ambulatory monitoring.

Hypertension: High blood pressure.

Hypotension: Low blood pressure.

Implantable cardioverter-defibrillator (ICD): An ICD is an automatic implanted electrical device used to detect and treat abnormal, fast heart rhythms. An ICD is usually implanted in the upper chest, and it performs cardioversion, defibrillation, and antitachycardia pacing.

Incompetence (valvular): Leakage through a heart valve; also referred to as *valvular insufficiency*.

Insufficiency (valvular): Leakage through a heart valve; also referred to as *valvular incompetence*.

Ischemia: The effect of insufficient blood flow to tissues due to lack of blood flow from blockage in the arterial system.

Lead: Also called an *electrode*. In an EKG machine or a pacemaker or an ICD system, it is the insulated wire or catheter that records electrical activity. A lead or electrode in a pacemaker or ICD conducts electrical energy from the device to the heart.

Left ventricular dysfunction: A heart condition in which the heart is unable to maintain normal cardiac output due to a muscular deficiency in the left ventricle.

Lipid: A fatty substance found in the blood.

Lipoprotein: A protein that carries lipids in the blood.

Magnetic resonance imaging (MRI): The use of a magnetic field and pulses of electromagnetic energy to make images of organs and structures inside the body.

Murmur: A sound made by blood flowing through a valve or a large blood vessel in the heart. A murmur may be normal or abnormal (see *bruit*).

Myocardial infarction: Death of a portion of the heart muscle tissue due to a blockage or interruption in the supply of blood to the heart muscle.

Myocardium: The middle and the thickest layer of the heart wall, which is composed of cardiac muscle.

Pacemaker: (A) Electrically active bundle of tissues in the heart that can spontaneously generate electrical impulses to make the heart beat. (B) An artificial device with a battery that generates regular electrical impulses to externally stimulate the heart to beat when it cannot do so on its own. Artificial pacemakers may be external and temporary, or implanted permanently into the chest wall.

Palpitation: A pounding painless but uncomfortable sensation felt in the chest due to an abnormal heartbeat.

Patent: Refers to a blood vessel that is still open, as opposed to being blocked, such as a *patent graft* or *patent ductus arteriosus*.

Percutaneous: The procedure of inserting a needle through the skin, often into an artery or a vein, so that a catheter can be delivered through the needle for diagnostic or treatment purposes.

Pericardium: The thin membrane that covers the heart.

Plaque: A collection of material often made of cholesterol, calcium, blood cells, and other material adhering to the wall of a blood vessel.

Pluripotent (stem cell): A stem cell that can develop in one of several ways—that is, become cells that can possibly turn into different cell types.

Premature atrial contraction (PAC): A contraction in the atrium, which is initiated by an ectopic focus and occurs earlier than the next expected normal sinus beat.

Premature ventricular contraction (PVC): A contraction in the ventricle started by an abnormal focus and that occurs earlier than the next expected normal sinus or rhythm beat.

Pulmonary: Pertaining to the lungs.

Pulmonary edema: Accumulation of fluid in the lungs, often due to heart failure, but may also be due to other causes.

Radiograph: The technical name of an X-ray image.

Radiography: The specialty dealing with imaging of the body by using X-rays.

Radioisotope: An isotope is a different version of the same element with a different atomic mass. If it is radioactive, with an unstable nucleus and the ability to emit radiation, the element is called a radioisotope.

Radionuclide: An atom with an unstable nucleus, which can undergo radioactive decay and emits ionizing radiation in the form of gamma rays and/or subatomic particles. Radionuclides occur naturally or can be artificially produced. They are used for producing radiologic images of internal organs.

Regurgitation: Backflow of blood through a valve that is opposite to the direction of normal flow.

Saphenous vein: A long vein that runs from the ankle to the groin that is used for coronary bypass grafting.

Septal defect: A hole in the septum that may be in the atrium (atrial septal defect) or in the ventricle (ventricular septal defect). Such defects are most often congenital but may occur due to damage from myocardial infarction.

Septum: The wall that separates the chambers of the heart. There are two septa in the human heart: the atrial septum and the ventricular septum.

Shunt: A connection between two blood vessels that is present at birth or surgically created.

Sinoatrial (SA) node: The heart's natural pacemaker located in the right atrium. Electrical impulses originate here and travel through the heart, causing it to beat regularly.

Stem cells: Cells that can divide and become differentiated into diverse specialized cell types and can also self-renew to produce more stem cells. In mammals, there are two types of stem cells: *embryonic* (isolated from a developing embryo) and *adult* (found in various tissues such as bone marrow).

Stenosis: Narrowing of a blood vessel or a valve that impedes flow of blood.

Stent: A device that is placed inside a blood vessel to prop it open, like a scaffolding.

Sternotomy: A cut in the sternum or breastbone to separate it in order to access the heart to perform heart massage or surgery.

Stroke volume: The amount of blood that is ejected by the left ventricle with each heartbeat, which is calculated by subtracting end-systolic volume (ESV) from end-diastolic volume (EDV).

Sudden cardiac death (SCD): Death due to cardiac causes within one hour of the onset of cardiac symptoms, and usually caused by ventricular fibrillation. In epidemiological studies, the term *sudden cardiac death* is also used to describe unwitnessed sudden death occurring in a presumably healthy person within a 24-hour period.

Supraventricular tachycardia (SVT): A tachycardia originating from above the ventricles. Also called *paroxysmal atrial tachycardia* (PAT).

Syncope: Fainting or loss of consciousness that may be due to a transient disturbance of cardiac rhythm (arrhythmia) or to other causes.

Tachyarrhythmia: Rapid beating of the heart over 100 beats per minute. There are atrial and ventricular tachyarrhythmias, depending on the site of origin.

Tachycardia (tachyarrhythmia): Rapid beating of either or both chambers of the heart, usually defined as a rate over 100 beats per minute.

Tamponade: The compression of the heart that occurs when fluid accumulates in the pericardial sac and prevents the heart from contracting normally.

Telemetry: The transmission of heart activity through radio waves from the patient to a monitor so that health professionals can observe the EKG of a patient 24 hours a day.

Thrombus: The technical name for a clot. When a clot detaches and travels to a remote location via the blood in the circulatory system, it is called an *embolus*.

Transvenous: Passage of an electrode or a probe through a vein after exposing or puncturing the vein.

Valve: A device that allows only one-way blood flow in the heart. There are four valves in the human heart.

Ventricle: One of the two lower pumping chambers of the heart (see *atrium*).

Ventricular fibrillation (VF): Very fast, chaotic, quivering heart contractions that start in the ventricles. During VF, the heart does not beat properly, resulting in cardiac arrest. Blood is not pumped from the heart to the rest of the body, and death will occur if defibrillation is not initiated within about six to ten minutes from the onset of VF.

Ventricular tachycardia (VT): A rapid heart rate that starts in the ventricles. During VT, the heart does not have time to fill with enough blood between heartbeats to supply the entire body with sufficient blood. It may cause dizziness light-headedness, fainting, and cardiac arrest.

USEFUL REFERENCES AND WEBSITES

Acierno, Louis J. *The History of Cardiology*. Pearl River, NY: Parthenon Publishing, 1994.
Fishman, Alfred P., and Dickinson, W. Richards, eds. *Circulation of the Blood: Men and Ideas*. New York: Oxford University Press, 1964.
Fuster, Valentin, Walsh, Richard, and Harrington, Robert. *Hurst's The Heart*, 13th ed. New York: McGraw-Hill, 2010.
Harvey, William. *On the Motion of the Heart and Blood*. Frankfurt, 1628 (Reprint).
Libby, Peter, Bonow, Robert O., Zipes, Douglas P., and Mann, Douglas L. *Braunwald's Heart Disease*, 8th ed. Philadelphia: Elsevier Health Sciences, 2007.

Websites

These websites provide detailed information on terms used in cardiology, specific diseases, treatment guidelines, dietary recommendations, consensus conferences, and how to find a cardiologist. A subscription is not necessary, but registration may be required.

American College of Cardiology: www.cardiosource.org
American Heart Association: www.heart.org
Centers for Disease Control and Prevention: www.cdc.gov
National Heart, Lung, and Blood Institute: www.nhlbi.nih.gov
National Library of Medicine: www.nlm.nih.gov

Index

About the Author

Dr. Regis A. DeSilva is associate professor of medicine at Harvard Medical School and a cardiologist at Beth Israel Deaconess Medical Center in Boston. After graduating from the Harvard Kennedy School of Government in 2004, he was director of Global Programs at Harvard Medical International, until 2011. Currently, he is also executive chairman of Global Medical Knowledge, Inc., which works in low-income and developing countries. He is, or has been, a Fellow of the Royal College of Physicians and Surgeons (Canada), a Fellow of the Royal Society of Medicine (United Kingdom), a Fellow of the American College of Cardiology, and president of the Boston Chapter of the American Heart Association. He lives in Cambridge, Massachusetts.